HEART MATTERS

A MEMOIR OF A FEMALE

HEART SURGEON

HEART MATTERS

Kathy E. Magliato, MD

Originally published as *Healing Hearts*

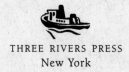

THREE RIVERS PRESS
New York

Over the years, I have treated many patients with heart disease. I am grateful to all of them for allowing me the opportunity to enter into their lives. All of the stories in this book are based on actual cases; however, in some of the examples I use, I have combined a number of elements, resulting in a composite of several individuals. And, of course, I have changed the names and distinguishing features of the men and women in this book in order to protect their privacy.

Originally published in hardcover as *Healing Hearts: A Memoir of a Female Heart Surgeon* in the United States by Broadway Books, an imprint of the Crown Publishing Group, a division of Random House, Inc., New York, in 2010.

Historical information in chapter 6 is taken from *The Story of Thoracic Surgery*, Andreas P. Naef (New York: Hans Huber Publishers, 1990).

Library of Congress Cataloging-in-Publication Data

Magliato, Kathy E.
Heart matters : a memoir of a female heart surgeon / Kathy Magliato.
p. cm.
1. Magliato, Kathy. 2. Heart surgeons—United States—Biography.
3. Women surgeons—United States—Biography. 4. Heart—Surgery—United States—Anecdotes. I. Title.

RD598.M165 2009
617.4'12092—dc22
[B]

2009033591

ISBN 978-0-7679-3027-7
eISBN 978-0-307-58919-4

Printed in the United States of America

Cover photograph by Kevin Foley

10 9 8 7 6 5 4 3 2 1

First Paperback Edition

To my sons, Gabriel and Nicholas, whose hugs and kisses
at the end of each challenging day heal *my* heart.

CONTENTS

HEART MATTERS

INTRODUCTION

Love at First Touch

IT WAS A CRAZY, HECTIC DAY. JUST LIKE ALL THE OTHERS.

People living. People dying. And there was much to do. There was blood to be drawn, labs to check, internal jugular lines to sink deep within a vein. There were Jackson Pratt drains to pull, notes to write, and discharge summaries to dictate. Rectal abcesses to I&D (incise and drain), wounds to clean and dress, and nasogastric tubes to insert into the nose and snake down the esophagus into the stomachs of patients with bowel obstructions without having it continually popping out the mouth or going up into the brain (I saw that once). There were patients piled knee-deep in the ER waiting to be seen and patients lined up around the block in admitting just waiting for a bed.

Where was I amid the chaos? I was standing in front of the operating room (OR) board, which displays all of the surgeries for the day. I was a general surgery intern and I had been up all night and was deliriously tired. I wasn't actually reading the OR board, just staring at it. Sleeping, if you will, with my eyes open. This is a trick I learned as a medical student during particularly long cases in which I had to stand frozen like a statue holding a retractor in order to give the operating surgeon exposure for some stupid gallbladder surgery. Whatever. I was jolted out of my stupor by a frantic nurse yelling, "Dr. Netter needs you stat in OR Seven!" Surely she wasn't talking to me. I was just a tired, depressed general surgery intern and Dr. Netter was a cardiothoracic surgeon. A big boy. Why would he need my help? I had never even scrubbed in on a cardiac surgery case and wouldn't know the first thing to do. Hell, I was so tired that, at one point, I couldn't remember if there were two hearts and one lung or one heart and two lungs in the thoracic cavity. While all of this was whizzing through my mind, the nurse grabbed me and dragged me to OR 7, opened the door, and threw me in. Like Kobe beef in a lion's den, I thought I'd be devoured whole. All hell was breaking loose inside and I hadn't a clue what to do. There was a lot of yelling. People were running around frantically. There was blood everywhere. It looked like Beirut. I tried not to slip and fall on my face in a pool of blood on my way to the OR table. One thing you need to know about blood is that it is as slippery as ice before it dries on an OR floor. I got within ten feet of the operating table, and without looking up, the surgeon (Dr. Netter, I presume, for I had never met the man) yelled, "Get some gloves on and get over here!" Get over where? By you, where all the blood is shooting up? "Oh, God," I thought, "the day is just beginning." I calmly (sort of) put on gloves and headed over to the table of horrors. Dr. Netter then said something that changed my life forever: "Grab the heart and hold it steady so I can get a few stitches in the hole we have here." As if "grab the heart" wasn't cool enough, he also said *we* as if he *and* I were part of this operation and would handle things together. When you're an intern and all you do is get yelled at and second-guessed and you live at the bottom of the surgical food chain, the word *we* by an attending feels pretty damn good in conjunction with anything related to surgery. I peered into the open chest cavity and there was the heart. Struggling to beat. Surrounded in a blood bath. It looked like a large, deformed matzo ball floating in tomato soup. I reached in and firmly yet gently closed my hand around the heart and around my future.

There is a myth that women make good surgeons because they have small, delicate hands. Nonsense. Mine are anything but petite. As a ten-year-old, I could palm a basketball, which somehow made me a popular pick for the basketball team in gym class even though palming a basketball has nothing to do with your ability to play the game. I could also hold down thirteen keys on the piano—a trait that led my mom to believe, incorrectly, that I would grow up to be a piano player, as she had. But here, in the OR, with a patient with a hole in his heart, a piano-key-spanning, basketball-palming, large-handed intern was *exactly* what Dr. Netter needed to save this patient's life. When I wrapped my hand around that heart, I could cradle it in just such a manner as to stabilize it perfectly for him to whip-stitch the hole shut.

Well, that was it for me. Love at first sight. Love at first touch. I knew that this was exactly what I wanted. To touch the human heart every day. It was the most amazing thing. The human heart. Firm and soft at the same time as it beat in my hand trying to get free of my grip.

When the heart muscle contracts, it becomes firm with the vigor of expelling blood with all its might. When the heart muscle relaxes, it softens and becomes flaccid to allow blood to gently flow into its chambers. Both functions are diametrically opposed and yet work in concert for one purpose and one purpose only—to sustain life.

And so I found myself holding this beautiful heart and being inspired. I asked Dr. Netter, "Do you do this every day?" "What?" he said, a little annoyed that I would be talking during such a critical time in the operation. "Touch the heart," I said. He looked up from what he was doing and, for the first time, made eye contact with me and said, "Of course I do! I'm a heart surgeon!" Then he just went back to saving the patient's life as if I had said nothing. My mind was reeling with the possibility that I could touch the human heart every day. What an incredible honor and privilege.

· · ·

This is my story. The story of a heart surgeon, wife, and mother trying to find a way to balance the toughness with the tenderness, the grief with the joy, the passion with the pain. Struggling every day to save lives. Struggling every day to achieve an equilibrium between my family and my career. Struggling every day to have it all and make a difference. Why do I struggle? Because there is no "app" for that.

This is their story. The story of women who have fought the good fight, most who ultimately succumbed to heart disease—a disease that is largely preventable. They will tell their story so that other women may learn from it and live.

This is our story. For my life and the lives of the women I am trying to save are forever intermingled.

1

Every Sixty Seconds

MAT: MAGLIATO-ADJUSTED TIME. IT'S GREENWICH MEAN time adjusted for the atomic clock plus twenty minutes. Which means it's your time plus twenty minutes. It's the clock I run on except, of course, when it's an emergency. Then I am there in a heartbeat (pun intended). Otherwise, it's whatever time you say you want me there—for dinner, for a playdate with the kids, for an eyebrow waxing—plus twenty minutes. And don't roll your eyes at me when I get there. You're lucky that I even showed up at all.

• • •

It was a still spring morning. The kind of morning that makes you *yearn* to be lazy. To languish in the comfort of your home while sipping coffee outside and smelling the morning ocean breeze of the Palisades, salt mixed with night-blooming jasmine. How I wish I could be lazy. Just once. When my alarm clock goes off at 5:03 a.m. (I always set it for an odd number), it's like a starter pistol for my day—assuming I ever went to sleep in the first place.

So I found myself that morning running on MAT. I desperately wanted to drop my son at school so I could maintain at least some semblance of motherhood. We were running late by everyone else's standards—twenty minutes late. I was surrounded by signs of road rage everywhere as I was trying to make my way safely to Nicholas's school. Everyone was on a cell phone, everyone was blowing a horn in a cacophony of rage, everyone was pissed off, everyone was yelling or gesturing to a neighboring car, and everyone was driving while intoxicated on Starbucks sugar-free vanilla lattes with regular milk. Yes, it was a typical three-mile commute to my son's school. My only hope was that there would be no accident so I would at least stand a chance of getting to school before they were singing the good-bye song under the good-bye tree. If there was to be a motor vehicle accident that day, perhaps it would be between two organ donors so that the whole day wouldn't be a wash.

I was making my way through an intersection on San Vicente Boulevard when a guy holding a cell phone under his chin, a coffee in his left hand, shifting with the right hand, driving with his knees while blowing his horn with his left elbow, and yes, folks, flipping another driver off with the middle finger of his free shifting hand nearly struck me. Multitasking at its best—and worst. I careened out of the way, missing him and the joggers and bicyclists along the side of the road (don't those people have jobs?). In the process, however, I spilled my coffee, which I had been balancing between my thighs (a trick my husband taught me), all over my lap. My entire car smelled like coffee and my thighs were on fire. Great. What else could go wrong today?

BEEP! BEEP! BEEP! BEEP! BEEP! BEEP! BEEP! BEEP!

It does that incessantly, you know, until you retrieve the page and turn it off. It's a sound that makes blood run from my ears. The first page of the day and it was from the cardiac catheterization lab, or cath lab as we call it, which is where patients get an angiogram to look for blockages in their coronary arteries. It is a place of pain and discovery for me and the patients. Thankfully, I was just pulling into the parking lot of the hospital when my pager went off.

The call was about a female pediatric patient who was having a heart attack. *Pediatric,* by my standards, is a patient in her thirties or forties, since most of our cardiac patients are well into their eighties and nineties. She was having a cardiac arrest, meaning that her heart had ceased to beat, and she was undergoing CPR. Any other information about her was irrelevant to me, including her name. I needed to get to the cath lab stat and further information over the phone would have just delayed me, as I can sprint from the parking lot faster with the phone on my belt clip than at my ear. Little did I know at the time that I would have the next three months to get to know everything about her and her family.

• • •

Dorothy was a vibrant forty-seven-year-old woman who successfully balanced raising six children while holding down a full-time job as a nurse for a gastroenterologist. She carried stress around like an American Express card. She never left home without it. It was her constant companion and she learned to just "live with it." It was simply woven into the fabric of her being.

For several months, she had been experiencing indigestion—a gnawing pain located in her upper abdomen, which was worsened by stress and relieved with rest at night. Recently, however, she was even waking at night with indigestion and kept a constant supply of antacids at her bedside, which she chewed like candy throughout the night. She told the gastroenterologist for whom she worked about her symptoms and he said, "It's probably an ulcer caused by stress. You should have an endoscopy to check it out." When all you have is a hammer, the whole world looks like a nail.

She was admitted to the hospital the following week for an upper gastrointestinal endoscopy—a simple outpatient procedure that uses a scope to look at the esophagus, stomach, and proximal small intestine. The gastroenterologist felt that as long as she was having an upper endoscopy, she might as well have a lower endoscopy, or colonoscopy, during the same appointment. It would be a waste of time and anesthesia not to check for colon cancer.

Her upper endoscopy was performed and found to be normal. Her lower endoscopy didn't go as smoothly. Inadvertently, her colon was perforated during the examination and a general surgeon was called to evaluate Dorothy. She required urgent surgery to repair the small hole in her colon. The abdominal surgery was straightforward and went well. Dorothy would make a full recovery and be out of the hospital in a few days. Or so she thought. But less than twelve hours later, while seeming to recover, Dorothy had a *massive* heart attack. She had the type of heart attack that, in medicine, we nickname "the widow maker" because it does one thing: It kills.

No one had bothered to ask Dorothy about her risk factors for heart disease. She had four. No one bothered to check her preprocedure EKG. It was abnormal. Why not? She was young. She was otherwise healthy. She was only having a "minor procedure" to look for an ulcer. But 1 in every 2.4 women will die from cardiovascular illness. Put another way, if you are reading this book and there is a woman seated on either side of you, look to your left. Look to your right. One and possibly two of you will succumb to heart disease. The American Heart Association estimates that one woman in the United States dies every sixty seconds from cardiovascular disease. In other words, the widow maker prefers women.

Dorothy was rushed to the cardiac catheterization lab for an emergency angiogram to evaluate the status of her coronary arteries—the arteries that bring life-giving blood to the heart. During an angiogram, dye is injected into the arteries and traces the path of blood flow. Like a road map, it reveals where the blockages are.

And there it was. The widow-maker lesion that causes a blockage in the main artery of the heart that essentially eliminates blood flow to the entire front and left side of the heart. Death takes on many forms, great and small. In this case, death was a three-millimeter collection of calcium, fat, and platelets beyond which no blood flowed.

By the time I arrived at the cath lab, Dorothy had arrested three more times. From the viewing room just outside the cath lab, I watched the team work to resuscitate her with the same efficiency as a NASCAR pit crew. Clear! Shock. Chest compressions. Adrenalin injection. Breathe. Repeat. And so the battle goes.

While I watched the resuscitation, I was faintly aware of two things: the pungent smell of the coffee I had spilled on my lap and the scent of charred flesh from the voltage being passed through her skin. The combination smelled like roasted marshmallows whose edges had been singed by a Lake George campfire.

The cardiologist who had performed the catheterization

approached me in haste. Sweat formed on his upper lip and brow. He had been working hard to save her.

"Is surgery an option here?" he said, his eyes drifting to my wet lap. I was accustomed to men addressing my breasts before, but this seemed *really* awkward. Then I remembered the coffee spill and realized he must think that I had wet myself in fear or that I have a serious incontinence issue. "Let's get this out of the way right now," I said, forcing eye contact. "I have not peed my pants in fear, and as long as we're on the subject of bodily fluids, I have never cried in the OR. It's spilled coffee. Now, to answer your question, yes, surgery is an option here. It's her only option." At this point it's fair to say that, in general, I can be a very blunt person. Comes with the territory.

The look of relief on his face changed his whole demeanor—from tense and apprehensive to relaxed and comfortable in his own skin again. Someone would save her when he couldn't. Medicine is always like this. We work as a team. We run a course of treatment, and when that course is exhausted and doesn't work, we hand the baton to another doctor with another course of treatment to run a different leg of the race to save a life. And we do this one life at a time.

It was while Dorothy's life hung delicately in the balance before my eyes that I decided that surgery was her only hope of survival. Without surgery, she would die. With surgery, she had a small chance. But it was better than no chance, and it was not time to give up. Not yet.

When it is my turn in the handoff to take the baton, I make a point to grab it with confidence and a firm grip. A feeble grip and a small measure of uncertainty can cause you to drop the baton and lose a patient's life. It can happen in a fraction of a second. I have found that you need to exude confidence to rally a team around a common goal, especially if most of the team feel that the effort involved in this leg of the race is futile. This was the case with Dorothy, as most of the nurses, technicians, and doctors in the room thought she was "too far gone."

With one hand I picked up the phone and called to the OR to get a room ready. With the other hand, I grasped the closest railing of the bed, unlocked the bed's brake with my foot, and started moving the patient single-handedly and single-mindedly toward the door of the cath lab.

"Pack her up, we're heading to the OR!" I called to the pit crew of nurses and techs.

Sometimes actions speak louder than words, and when they saw me start moving the bed, they were on board with my plan. As I said: firm grip, confidence.

The team knew exactly what to do. Someone took over the ambu bag and squeezed it to breathe for Dorothy while we transported her. Another tech threw the portable monitors, IV bags, and tubing as well as the defibrillator onto the moving bed. We looked like quite the parade moving down the hallway with calculated speed.

We brought her to the operating room with me riding on the gurney straddling her waist and performing chest compressions. My strategy to save her life was this: I would open her chest and try to restart her arrested heart by methodically squeezing it with my hands—a technique known as open heart massage. If I got her back, I would operate. If not, I would let her die. It was very binary—a "go" or "no-go" decision. Surgeons make these decisions all the time. It is part of the fabric that we are made of.

We entered the operating room, and despite the fact that the temperature in the OR was 55 degrees (I like a frigid operating room), we were all sweating. Maybe it was the adrenaline rush of saving a life, maybe it was simply the trip there, but either way, we all looked like we had just finished a marathon. However, the tough part of this race was about to begin.

We moved her to the operating table.

"Okay, people, on my count. Ready? On three . . . Three!"

Yes, we skip the one and the two. Who has time for that? Only on TV do they bother with the whole one-two-three thing.

During this whole process of moving Dorothy from the gurney to the OR table, by the way, I am trying to maintain an air of calm while in my head I am quietly rehearsing the ten thousand moves it will take me to perform this woman's bypass surgery. All the while I am continuing to do chest compressions. The nurses begin to "prep me into the wound," which means they pour Betadine, a dark bronze-colored skin cleansing agent, all over my hands, wrists, and forearms as well as the patient's chest. It makes me look like I have just dipped my hands into a barrel of maple syrup up to my elbows. The nurses then drape the patient with sterile linens while bringing the drapes around my body so as not to drape me into the sterile field. Once the draping is done, I allow someone else who is now wearing sterile gloves to take over compressions while I run to the scrub sink to formally prep my hands.

I reentered the operating room to find that Dorothy still had no spontaneous heartbeat. I quickly opened her chest using a No. 10 blade Bard-Parker scalpel—your standard-issue scalpel. Scalpels come in all shapes and sizes. Straight. Curved. Wide. Thin. They all have one thing in common, though, which is that with very little pressure they can slice through skin, collagen, and muscle like butter. I made an incision down the middle of Dorothy's sternum that was much larger than I normally make. I needed maximum exposure to her heart. If this were a breezy, nonchalant, elective surgery on a rainy afternoon, I would cut through only the most superficial layer of skin, the epidermis, so as not to cause much bleeding. Just capillary bleeding at the skin edge. But because during the time I was opening Dorothy's chest she would have no chest compressions and therefore no blood flow to her brain and other vital organs, speed was essential. I applied a healthy pressure to the scalpel handle and cut her to the bone with one swipe of the knife. I ignored the flood of blood into the field and had my assistant suction it out of the way as if it were simply a nuisance and not the precious commodity that it is. I used a handheld sternal saw with a blade that oscillates up and down to open her breastbone from the notch at the base of the neck below the Adam's apple to the xiphoid process at the midpoint of the upper abdomen. My assistant and I each took an edge of sternum and pulled toward ourselves using our body weight as countertraction. Like breaking a wishbone, we pulled her sternum apart and placed a retractor along the sternal edge to hold the chest open.

I immediately reached in and began open cardiac massage by gently pushing down on her heart, which was covered by a sac called the pericardium and mediastinal fat, which is a remnant of the thymus gland. Pushing down forces the heart to eject blood from both ventricles, or lower chambers. When you release the pressure, you allow the heart to passively fill. Push down. Let up. Push down. Let up. Sounds easy, but it's not. I've seen surgeons, in the heat of the moment, put their finger right through the heart.

Here, incidentally, would be a good point to tell you about the nuances of open versus closed cardiac massage should you find yourself at a near-fatal auto accident with a scalpel and sternal saw at your disposal. Closed cardiac massage, in which you push down on the patient's sternum in an effort to compress the heart between the breastbone and the backbone, requires vigorous effort, as you need to depress the sternum by about four to five centimeters. Too light a touch and you won't get adequate compressions to cause the heart to expel blood. Too vigorous and you break ribs and puncture lungs, which does more harm than good. When I was a medical student, I was told that "if you're not breaking ribs, you're not doing it right." Macabre medical humor noir, maybe, but the first time I did CPR as a medical student it was on an old man and I swear with my first compression I heard (and felt!) every rib snap like dry twigs underfoot. *Eeeeew!* You have no idea how grotesque that is. Open cardiac massage on the other hand is done with a firm but light touch like squeezing one of those "stress balls" in the palm of your hand. Great care is essential because you can, quite literally, rip a heart in two with your gloved hands.

After opening the pericardial sac, I was able to restart Dorothy's heart by using a combination of internal defibrillation, in which we apply electricity-generating paddles directly on the surface of the heart to send a current through the heart itself, and injections of Adrenalin directly into the heart muscle. It may seem harsh, but we are trying to save a life here. Next, I proceeded with a double bypass operation to reroute blood around the widow-maker blockage and restore blood flow to the front and left side of her heart. The surgery went surprisingly well. Dorothy left the operating room in stable but critical condition. But would her body and mind recover from such a profound insult? Only time would tell.

For the first few days she appeared to stabilize and do well. She awakened after two days of deep sedation and was able to communicate. Even though she remained on a ventilator and unable to speak, she "spoke" with those around her by nods and gestures. This, in itself, was nothing short of a miracle because when the heart is arrested, there is no blood flow to the brain and I half expected her not to regain consciousness at all. I spoke to her and told her what had happened and that it was amazing that she was even alive. She rolled her eyes and gestured with the palm of her hand on her forehead in an "I could've had a V8" mannerism as if to say that she knew she was in this predicament because she (and, sadly, her doctors) ignored the warning signs.

I admit now that I was lulled into a false sense of security because she just "looked so good." The first sign that something was amiss was a decrease in her urine output. The kidneys are like a canary in a coal mine. In general, they will be the first to alert you that there is something gravely wrong with the body. We like to see a urine production of one milliliter per kilogram of weight per hour. So for a seventy-kilogram (154-pound) woman, we expect seventy milliliters of urine per hour. Short of that, you start to look for causes of low urine output because you only have a short period of time to rectify the situation before the kidneys shut down and dialysis ensues. The kidneys, by the way, annoy me. They are so fickle and demanding. The slightest drop in blood perfusion to the kidney and they get pissed off (pun intended, again) and quit working. What babies! Then you have to coddle them back into working again, all the while you know they have the upper hand because without them you're toast.

Inevitably, as often happens to someone whose heart has stopped too long, Dorothy didn't do so well. One complication after another attacked her body, slowly eliminating her organ function like shooting ducks at an arcade. First the kidneys, then the lungs, then the liver, and so on. Dominoes waiting to topple. The process, known as multisystem organ failure, is lethal. The coup de grâce was an infection that set up camp in her bloodstream, sending tiny bacterial soldiers out on a search-and-destroy mission to invade every remote location of her body. This is called sepsis. It is yet another form that death can take.

After three months of battle, months where she lapsed into and out of consciousness, months that we hoped weren't lived in pain, the family felt that it was time to surrender. They had lingered at her bedside every day. They had watched her fluctuate between good days, when she seemed to brighten up, and bad days, when her color would turn milky gray and she was essentially unresponsive to their gentle stroking. They had watched her undergo a plethora of procedures to sustain her life—tracheostomy, dialysis catheter, stomach feeding tube, indwelling venous lines. When they approached me one morning to tell me it was "time," I already knew what they were going to say before they mouthed the actual words. It was as if somewhere for them a clock had stopped. I could see it in their sullen eyes, their stooped posture, their wringing hands. I can always tell when a family is ready to let go. I am fully fluent in body language.

Such a lovely, compassionate family who remained so supportive of me and my efforts throughout those three months. We had all simultaneously come to the same conclusion—that our greatest weapon, hope, was gone. There was no hope that

Dorothy would make a full recovery. It is always hard for me to accept this moment. The moment when we give up. Something in me has to die in order for me to let go. Some essence of hope that I hold dear has to leave me and die. I must always respect the wishes of a patient's family, though, because I know, in my heart, that they understand what the patient would want at this juncture better than I ever could. I have to trust them. I have to. I see patients live who should die and I see patients die who should live, but it is not for me to judge the situation so I must simply lay down my weapons of healing and trust the family.

As the family and I gathered around Dorothy's bedside, we began the process of disconnecting her from life support. I first moved all of the extraneous equipment out of the room so the family could have 360-degree uncluttered access to Dorothy's body to touch her and kiss her whenever and wherever they wished. I brought down the bed rails and encouraged them to get into bed with her and hold her, which a few of her children did. We pulled out her nasogastric tube, which had been inserted into her right nostril and snaked into her stomach when her PEG tube (a percutaneous endoscopic gastrostomy feeding tube inserted directly into the stomach through the abdominal wall) malfunctioned, so that her face was free of any medical-looking paraphernalia. She appeared human again. We made her comfortable by infusing a continuous drip of morphine, which we titrated as needed. We turned off the alarms on all of the monitors so as her blood pressure and heart rate softened, the family would not be jolted by an ear-piercing alarm that screams at everyone in the room, "I am dying! I am dying! Can't you see?" We disconnected her from the dialysis machine but not the ventilator because I thought it might be uncomfortable for her to try to breathe on her own. Last, we turned off the medications that were supporting her blood pressure, the tube feedings, and all other medications except the morphine drip.

I shut the outer door of her private ICU room to muffle any sound from other patients and staff in the unit. The only sound in the room was the whoosh of the ventilator that seems to whisper *iiiiiinnnnn, ooooouuuuuttttt*. In fact, if you say the word *in* while you are inhaling and say *out* while you are exhaling, it is exactly what a ventilator sounds like. Other than the ventilator, the only other sound in Dorothy's room was soft sobbing. Mine and theirs.

• • •

In the end, how long do you think it took Dorothy to die once she was disconnected from life support? It took sixty seconds. And, yes, it may have taken her three months to get to those sixty seconds, but in the end, death came within sixty seconds. So when I say that a woman dies every sixty seconds from heart disease, it may just be the most horrific sixty seconds of her life and her family members' lives.

2

The Persistent Heart

THE HUMAN HEART. IT IS A THING OF BEAUTY AND AWE. Like snowflakes, no two hearts are alike. One may be stout and strong while another is weak and frail. Each heart has subtle differences in its anatomy, coloration, sphericity, and positioning in the chest. But they all have one thing in common—persistence. It is the one word that I feel best describes the heart. When the human heart is cut from the chest of a patient about to receive a fresh transplant, it will continue to beat in the specimen tray in which it is placed for several minutes before it finally comes to rest. Like a freshly caught fish on the deck of a boat, the heart doesn't know that it has been snatched from the chest and continues to wriggle with life.

The average heart beats eighty times per minute, which means that, in any given day, your heart will beat approximately one hundred thousand times. In a year it will have beaten forty-two million times and in a lifetime it will beat nearly three billion times. All the while, it is taking in blood and expelling it to the lungs and throughout the body. The heart pumps approximately one million barrels of blood in a lifetime, which equals the capacity of three supertankers. It does not rest. It does not tire. It is persistent in its drive and purpose. Yes. It is an object of beauty and awe.

The heart is also the great equalizer. It levels the playing field between women and men. I am often asked to describe the difference between a man's heart and a women's heart. I smirk when I get this question because inside the chest cavity, we are the same, men and women. Men's hearts are neither stronger nor greater than women's hearts. True, women's hearts tend to be smaller, and perhaps the tissues are a bit more delicate, but a woman's heart is no less mighty than a man's. They are equally persistent.

Likewise, if you take two people of different race and cover them completely with sterile drapes, I cannot tell if they are African American, Caucasian, Asian, or Hispanic by looking at their hearts. Discrimination is an external phenomenon. On the inside, we are all equal.

And yet, despite the fact that we are all equal on the inside, death from cardiovascular disease is discriminatory against women because it has killed more women than men every year since 1985! Cardiovascular disease attacks the hearts of women and kills in epidemic proportions. It is a misogynist.

It also discriminates against African Americans because they are at higher risk for heart disease and stroke than Caucasians. In fact, the age-adjusted rate of heart disease for African American women is 72 percent higher than for white women. Yes, we are all alike and then again we are not.

• • •

Journeying inside the thoracic cavity to behold the human heart is no easy feat but most certainly worth the effort. After all, our entire chest cavity—the sternum or breastbone in front, the ribs along our sides and thoracic spine along our back—was designed to protect our most vital organ. These bony structures form a fortress or cage (as in rib cage) to house and secure our precious treasure. Forget about the lungs. We have two of those. We could misplace one or shish-kebab one with a spear and it would be no big deal. But the heart, in its singular beauty, is infinitely more vital. I am in-different to lungs unless, of course, I am resecting a cancer that has taken up residence in its tissues. I acknowledge their presence in the thoracic cavity, but frankly, they take up too much space and just get in my way.

Entering the thoracic cavity takes skill and upper body strength. I once saw a cardiac surgeon zip open a chest and, in the process, cut the heart clean in two with the sternal saw. Very messy. Blood shot out of the chest, hit the operat-ing table lights, and dripped down on the backs of our necks for the remainder of the case, which lasted another three minutes until the patient bled to death. That's why I listed skill first and strength second.

There is a ceremonious preparation that occurs before a patient's chest is opened. One must first don the appropriate garb—headdress and all—engage in the cleansing ritual, and finally, identify the appropriate "opening music"—the special songs that all heart surgeons like to listen to while opening the chest. For me it is always R&R. Yes, good old rock and roll and not the crap that is now being passed off as rock and roll. Anything from AC/DC to Zeppelin. Oh, sure, I listen to my high school oldies like Meat Loaf, REO Speedwagon, and

Journey and then sometimes resort to Social Distortion to appease my perfusionist, Steve (more about perfusionists later). For the more mellow parts of the surgery, which require slower moves, it's Sting, Dido, Annie Lennox, and Pink Floyd. Nothing is so relaxing as taking down an internal mammary artery to "Dark Side of the Moon."

There are two very important things I do before I begin any operation: I pee and I eat. Why? Because I never know when I will have a chance to do either of these two things again. Think of the OR as a vortex. It sucks you in and when you are inside, spinning, time stops. I have stood for eighteen hours in an operating room, which is to say that I have just as much, if not more, endurance than most male surgeons, and a bigger bladder. I am so focused during an operation that I can put my head down and stare into a six-by-ten-inch hole in the chest starting at 7:00 a.m. until I next pick my head up and glance at the clock, when it is "suddenly" 2:30 or 4:30 or 8:30 p.m. And I have no idea how the time flew by.

So after the quick trip to the bathroom and the downing of four ounces of low-fat cottage cheese (a staple for me), I proceed with getting dressed for the occasion. I wear a headlight like a miner's headlight only smaller. The purpose of it is twofold: It gives me added light, which I use to focus on the operative field, and, more important, it signifies who the lead surgeon is. The alpha male or, in this case, the alpha female. The headlight is tightened around my head and rests at the level on my midforehead. If it's too tight it will bore a hole through your skull. I, by the way, have a subtle dent in my forehead (which I plan to fill in with collagen as soon as I have a moment) from a twelve-hour seven-vessel reoperative bypass case I did a few months ago. The surgery was so difficult and intense that I didn't feel the headlight pressing on my skull and causing a necrosis of my subdermal tissue. Yes, I am very focused in the OR.

After the headlight, I put on specialized glasses called loupes, which magnify everything in their field 3.5 times. These enable me to sew one-millimeter-diameter vessels together with thread (called suture) that is finer than a human hair. They are customized to my interpupillary distance and my focal length (the distance from my eyes to where my hands rest during surgery). With the headlight and my glasses, I am carrying a few pounds on my head during surgery, which wreaks havoc on my neck and back, and because of this I am now incapable of turning my neck a full 180 degrees from side to side. That is why you see most heart surgeons with a stooped posture and a jutting chin. It's a telltale sign of our profession. Just attend one of our surgical conventions—we look like a bunch of Nixons milling about.

After the donning of the headdress along with a surgical cap and mask that altogether ruin your hair, I then need to scrub my hands, wrists, and forearms in a traditional manner that has been handed down from surgeon to surgeon. I was taught how to scrub properly as a medical student, and if I didn't get it right they made me start all over again. No one keeps surveillance on me now; we use the honor system. The entire process takes seven minutes and we use a special scrub brush that has a sponge on one side and a plastic brush on the other. We must meticulously scrub our nails and nail beds, since that is where most of the bacteria hide. I have always dreamed of having long luxurious nails but, alas, surgeons must cut their nails to the quick with only a thin edge of white showing. No nail polish. Ever. Someday, I would like to put on long acrylic nails, paint them a vamp red, and waltz into the OR just to see if the scrub nurse would glove me with those daggers on. Hey, I see women with nails like that who type and work a cash register. Why not heart surgery? One can always dream.

After scrubbing for surgery, I dry my hands completely with a sterile towel handed to me by the scrub nurse, who is already scrubbed and dressed in sterile garb. Since they no longer make surgical gloves with powder inside, if your hands are even slightly wet, you have a tough time slipping them into the gloves. This is a key maneuver because it's sexy to glide into a pair of sterile gloves that *snap!* onto your hands. It makes you feel like a slick surgeon, master of your domain. If you fumble with wet hands you look like a dunce and everyone in the room thinks you're a hack. First impressions are crucial.

Then, on goes the gown, tied in the back by a nonsterile nurse called a circulating nurse. You must spin, release your end of the waist tie to the nurse, and deftly tie it at your side. All the while you are trying not to bump into anything, which might contaminate you, in which case you'd have to start all over again. You have no idea the number of times I screwed up the routine as a medical student before I could do it in one take. And we haven't even gotten to the operation yet . . .

As the lead surgeon (with the headlight and all) I move to the surgeon's side of the operating table. This is always at the patient's right side. My assistant stands at the left side. Now for you lefties out there—and my husband is one— *tough*. You have to operate from the patient's right even though it would be easier for you to operate from the left. Why? Good ol' boy tradition. You look like a sissy operating from the left. Everyone will think you are the lowly assistant even if you do wear the headlight headdress. Get over it. They all do. This club has tough rules.

The surgery begins with the opening of the skin that covers the chest. I am compulsive about making my incision perfectly in the midline of the chest. At times, I will mark the center of the sternum in two places and use a string to draw a straight line between the two points. Other times I simply eyeball it, using what I consider to be my uncanny knack for being able to judge, with near perfect accuracy, when something is straight and level (which, incidentally, is why I drive my husband crazy when he tries to hang a picture on the wall in our home). Here's the deal: If what you see on the outside is perfect and straight, you can assume that the work done on the inside is equally as good. And, for those of you ladies who have had your breasts "enhanced," I am quite the pro at being able to make an incision exactly between them so as not to pop your implants.

When I am ready to cut, I will call out "incision!" as I lay the scalpel to the skin to notify the anesthesiologist that I am making the incision. They record this time in the OR record and anesthesia record. Once inside the chest, after the heart is exposed, I have this secret little tradition/ritual that I do. I touch the heart first, before my assistant does. Just a little light stroke with my finger tip or knuckle. So subtle a move that no one has ever noticed and I have never told anyone about it until now. Why? Because I want to be the first. *I* opened the door to the secret chamber that houses the heart and *I* want to be the first to touch it. Neil Armstrong got to be the first one to touch the moon. Maybe that was prearranged by NASA. Or maybe, just maybe, he was simply the first one at the door.

After tickling the heart, my next job is to "get on pump," which is heart-surgeon-speak for establishing a connection between the patient and the heart-lung machine, which circulates the patient's blood outside the body and gives it oxygen. This is done so that the heart can be at rest and those pesky lungs can remain deflated and out of my way. The steps to get on pump are written in stone and every surgeon has his or her own stone. In other words, the basic steps to get on pump are the same for every heart surgeon, but each will have her or his subtle, but just as unwavering, differences. These steps must be memorized by everyone in the room or the personal cadence of the moves is ruined, pissing the surgeon off.

Heparin, a powerful blood thinner made from cow lung or pig intestine (seriously), is administered intravenously. This enables blood to spin through the heart-lung machine without clotting. Next a sequence of special stitches known as purse-string sutures are placed into the aorta and the right upper chamber of the heart (the atrium). They are called purse-string sutures because, when you pull up on them, they gather up the tissue trapped in the center of the suture. Through the center of these sutures I pass a cannula, which is a large-bore tube made of special plastic that will direct blood out of the body, to the pump, and back to the body again. I secure each cannula in place using the purse-string sutures, de-air it (if air gets into the system and is pumped to the patient, it causes a massive stroke from an air embolism), and then connect the cannula to the bypass circuit tubing. When this procedure is complete, I note this by announcing to the entire staff in the room that I am ready to "go on pump." At each step in this sequence, communicating to the team is key.

The most important team member in the room, by the way, is not, as you might think, my surgical assistant but rather the perfusionist. A perfusionist is the person who runs the heart-lung machine—my wingman or wingwoman. They watch my back (literally, because they are positioned behind me in the OR) and keep me flying a straight course through to a successful surgery, or "pump run," as we call it. We have a symbiotic relationship for we cannot exist without each other. On a personal note, I have always considered the perfusionists with whom I have worked among my dearest friends. Navigating through death and back brings us closer. That, and the fact that they are a great bunch of guys (and girls!) who are, by far, the coolest people in the room. It is unfortunate, in my opinion, that they seem to get very little credit for the success of an operation even though they are integral to it. Most people undergoing heart surgery don't even know perfusionists exist. They think the heart-lung machine just "runs by itself." The next time you have heart surgery, it would be nice if you baked your perfusionist some brownies as a gesture of thanks because the bottom line on the heart-lung machine is that if a perfusionist and I put you "on pump" and can't get you off at the end of the case, you're a dead woman.

• • •

Once I have the patient on the heart-lung machine, I drain all the blood from her heart so that it is fully decompressed. In this flaccid, baggy state, the heart is yielding. It is easy to manipulate and position to achieve the best exposure to the area upon which I need to operate. I feel sorry for the heart in this state. It is vulnerable and only a shell of its former mighty beating self. I can have my way with a heart in this decompressed state because it submits to my will. This, however, just doesn't seem right even though I have put the heart in this state so I can fix it. Sometimes we must yield control to others and accept our vulnerability so we can be healed.

The last step in having total control over the heart is to shut it down or arrest it. This is done by administering a high-potassium solution known as cardioplegia directly into the coronary arteries. We also place ice slush on the heart to cool it topically while simultaneously cooling the patient's body temperature to 28 to 32 degrees C. Creating a "heart snow cone" is important because by cooling the heart, we decrease its metabolism and this allows us to preserve the heart's function while at rest.

The heart at rest looks so unnatural. It is, after all, what death looks like, because only in death do our hearts cease to beat. Performing heart surgery, therefore, is all about taking a patient, in a controlled state, to the brink of death and back to life again. It is a very privileged journey that only heart surgeons get to take on a daily basis. For us, it is routine. Ho hum. As in "What did you do at work today, honey?" "Oh, I stopped someone's heart and then brought them back to life." And yes, it is pretty damn cool. It beats brain surgery hands down. Why? Because in the majority of cases, all brain surgeons do is "suck the brain." They are not sewing one-millimeter vessels together with their bare (okay, gloved) hands. Instead, they take suction catheters and vacuum out tumors while leaving behind normal brain tissue. I would like to see a neurosurgeon go home, open up the refrigerator, take out some cooked angel hair pasta (overcooked, not al dente) and sew the ends together with a thread the size of a strand of human hair—because that's what it is like to do bypass surgery.

Once the heart is stopped I must work quickly to perform whatever reparative surgery I need to do, be it coronary artery bypass grafting, valve repair or replacement, ablation of an abnormal rhythm pattern, or repair of a tear in the aorta. There is a limit to how long the heart and body can withstand being on the heart-lung machine. After approximately four hours or so, the more fickle end organs, such as the lungs, brain, kidneys, and liver, suffer damage. Also, the longer you are on pump, the more difficult it is to restart the heart. As with many things in life that require certain risks, there is an envelope here that can be pushed. But you can push this particular time envelope just so far, because hitting the point of no return literally means the patient leaves the OR in a body bag. Sound judgment, combined with alacrity and skill, must always prevail in a heart surgeon's operating theater.

Once the surgery is complete, the perfusionist and I go through the process of restarting the heart and weaning the patient from the heart-lung machine. We begin by rewarming the patient to a near-normal body temperature. We cease the administration of the cardioplegia solution that is paralyzing the heart and, instead, perfuse the heart with the patient's warmed blood. Then we watch and we wait. It doesn't take long for the heart to stir. Like a young child waking up from a long afternoon nap, the heart will beat for a moment, then fall back to "sleep," only to stir and beat again intermittently when ready. Often, we have to coax it back into beating by shocking it with a low level of voltage from an internal defibrillator paddle. I always hate doing this because it seems like such a rude thing to do to the heart (can you imagine waking your toddler up with a cattle prod?). I much prefer to take a more patient stance and allow the heart to wake up on its own volition. When the heart is beating in a normal rhythm, we proceed to wean the patient from the heart-lung machine. This is done by gradually decreasing the amount of blood pumped by the machine while simultaneously increasing the amount of blood being pumped by the heart. This is the most crucial time of the surgery because how well a patient comes "off pump" tells us a lot about how well the patient will do after the surgery is over. The coordination between the surgeon and her wingman, the perfusionist, is paramount for a successful weaning and separation to occur. Like cutting an umbilical cord, there is always an exact moment of separation and, within that moment, a brief, almost fleeting uncertainty of whether or not a patient will "fly off pump," meaning that she will survive the process. It is a lot to ask of the heart to suddenly take up its responsibility to beat and pump blood again once it has tasted the sweet serenity of being at rest because, unless you have had heart surgery before, your persistent heart has *never* rested in your lifetime.

After all this drama, closing the patient up is a piece of cake. As with opening music, I have closing music, which is always the B-52s. Rock on. The heart-lung machine cannulas are removed, and the heparin given to thin the blood is reversed with a drug called protamine, which is made from salmon sperm (no kidding). When the blood starts to clot again and there is no more bleeding (a process called "achieving hemostasis"), two large drains called chest tubes are placed in the chest. The chest tubes will exit out the front of the upper abdomen and will drain any further bleeding after surgery. The breastbone is wired back together using heavy stainless-steel wires that are permanent and the skin is closed in three layers of dissolvable suture. Voilà! My patient has now joined the "zipper club" and will forever wear that scar as a badge of courage. A scar that is as persistent as the heart itself. A scar of survival.

3

Oh, Nurse!

THE BIRTH OF A SURGEON

"Who the hell are you, my nurse?"

"I'm the heart surgeon who is going to operate on you."

"Like hell you are! You don't look like a heart surgeon."

"How is a surgeon supposed to look?"

"Well, I'd expect you to be older, have your hair in a bun, and wear glasses."

"That would be the librarian," I say, rolling my eyes and exiting the room.

THE YEAR WAS 1999. IT WAS MY FIRST DAY AS AN ATTENDing staff cardiothoracic surgeon and I wasn't about to take any shit from anyone. If I had a dollar for every time someone mistook me for a nurse, I'd be a very rich woman by now and wouldn't have had to go through the grueling training of a cardiac surgeon. All I could think about as I exited this man's room was that it was going to be all uphill from here. But it had *already been* an uphill journey to becoming a heart surgeon, and boy, was I tired! The odd thing was, to the contrary, that my most vivid memory of how that journey began was with a gentle push downhill.

• • •

The fondest memory of my childhood was not making snow angels in the crusty winters of upstate New York or ice-skating in Sixteenth Woods, a swamp on our farm. Nor was it jumping into a pile of musty brown-orange-red leaves in the fall. It wasn't eating the nectar of honeysuckle or the arrival of the magnolia blossoms in spring. No, it wasn't even hiking Mohonk Mountain with Aunt Evie in summer, our backpacks laden with hero sandwiches and Yoo-Hoos from Bordi's Deli.

My fondest memory of childhood was the day my grandfather took off my training wheels. "Poppop," as we called him, was my mom's father. He and Nana (my mom's mother) lived next door to us. They were German immigrants who came to the United States by way of Ellis Island in 1921 at the tender ages of seventeen and sixteen, respectively.

When Poppop gripped your hand, you could see the muscles of his forearm bulge and his hand, the coarse hand of a worker, would envelop your own. He'd always say to me, "You can tell the character of a person by their handshake." I can close my eyes and see him saying this with his toothy, sincere smile and earnest eyes. He still is, to this day, the most trustworthy man I have ever met. What I loved best about him, though, was that he always smelled like wood chips and I could invariably find him by going to the basement of his house, where he tinkered in his workshop while listening to John Philip Sousa.

I remember the morning that he marched across the yard, wrench in hand, and took off my training wheels without saying a word. We lived in a modest house that my parents built (I have pictures of my very pregnant mother on a ladder painting it!) in the quaint town (actually called a village) of Highland, New York, in the Hudson River valley. Most people look at me quizzically when I say that I am from High-land because most people have never heard of the place and we Highlanders like our anonymity. So I usually give people general clues as to its whereabouts: It's somewhere between West Point Military Academy and the CIA (Culinary Institute of America). Have you seen the movie *The French Connection*? Remember the part where Gene Hackman, interrogating a sus-pect while wearing a Santa Claus suit, says, "Do you pick your feet in Poughkeepsie?" Highland's on the other side of the Hudson River from that. Ever been to Woodstock? You know, Yasqur's farm, hippies, flower power? We're near there.

Highland is a place where business is still done on a hand-shake. Where people leave their homes unlocked at night and their keys in the car at the grocery store—or anywhere, for that matter. It's where my favorite local police officer's last name is Sargent, giving him the distinction of being addressed as "Sergeant Sargent" and who bear-hugs me, sidearm and all, every time I see him. It's a place where the Lombardi sisters, who are well into their eighties, will bake a lemon cake for you the size of a tire and drop it by your house at eight o'clock in the morning just because you are in visiting from California. For me, it was a place to stay and leave all at the same time. I certainly didn't appreciate its beauty and homespun kindness while growing up there. No, I certainly didn't. And now, for me, that beauty and kindness is something I couldn't live with-out because it grounds me somehow.

We lived on a hill and my grandfather took me to the top of the incline and told me to ride down the road. When I told him that I was afraid, he said, "Don't worry, *schatzi* [his nick-name for me, which means "sweetheart" in German], I'll be right behind you all the way, holding on to your seat." I started pedaling down that hill, faster and faster I went without so much as a wobble. I marveled at my speed and thought, "Gee, I can't believe how fast Poppop can run!" About halfway down, I looked back and saw that marvelous grin beaming at me from the top of the hill, his hands resting on his hips.

My whole life has been like that. Anything that I have ever accomplished has been with my family, an invisible hand, balancing me, supporting me, pushing me forward. My parents, my siblings, and later my husband and children, are always behind me as I pedal up and down life's hills. ·

To say that my childhood was filled with bike rides and endless frolicking would be very, very far from the truth. We lived on a fifty-acre apple orchard and that meant one thing— work. Sure, the orchard was a great place to run in the tall grass, catch voles, and sit up in the cherry trees and eat dead-ripe cherries, pits and all, until you were sick. It was also a swell place to have apple fights with your brothers, using wooden crates as bunkers and rotten apples as ammo. Yes, it was great for all that, but we spent far more time working in that orchard than playing in it.

Despite the fact that my dad had a steady job working at IBM, we never seemed to have enough money to support ourselves. I grew up thinking that milk came only in powdered form. That everyone buys their clothes at the hardware store and that setting the thermostat at 58 degrees F in winter was "warm enough." When we had no money for meat because it was "expensive," my mom made "gravy bread," which was a piece of bread with gravy on it. When we had no money to pay our utilities, my mother would put the phone bill check in the oil bill envelope and vice versa. By the time the utility companies straightened out the error, my dad would have another paycheck.

I never really felt poor, though, because what we lacked

around our home was made up for in love and an unfailing pride instilled in us by our parents. The only time I ever felt ashamed about our lack of funds was at the grocery checkout when my mother would look at the running total with increasing worry. Inevitably, we would have to put items back because we had come up short, so my mom would use us as "runners" to bring the groceries back to their rightful aisle. I just hated that pitiful look from the people in line behind us.

And so that it is how it came to pass that we, the children, farmed the orchard for additional income. We set aside several acres of land for vegetables and grew corn, tomatoes, peppers, potatoes, zucchini, pumpkins, carrots—whatever my father's whim was at the time. He was one tough cookie and a disciplinarian who believed that hard work paid off. One year he decided to plant *three thousand* tomato plants. We thought we would die. There was no playing after school. Just work. Berry-hooking. Weeding. Fertilizing. My dad (now, I know this is going to sound crazy) had us carry around old Maxwell House coffee cans half full of gasoline into which we would drop Japanese potato beetles plucked from the potato plants. Hadn't he ever heard of pesticides? Oh, that would probably have cost too much money.

When the vegetables were harvested, we would sit in our garage until the wee hours of the morning and "shine" them, polishing the dirt off them with a soft cloth and neatly stacking them in bushel baskets. Then, before school, my mother would drive us to the farmers' market to sell the fruits (and vegetables) of our labor. To this day, I have no idea how I graduated at the top of my high school class. When did I have time to study?

One would think that during the winter months in New

York we would have a reprieve from farming chores. Not a chance. In the winter, we would shovel driveways for cash. My parents saved our earnings for us, and when we had enough money, we bought a snow plow for our farming tractor. One of my brothers drove the farm tractor (with no cab on it, mind you) and plowed the driveways while my sister and I shoveled the customers' sidewalks for an extra two dollars. Eventually, we had enough for a pickup truck and my brothers used it to haul salt and coarse sand to spread on the driveways and side-walks. During the nonwinter months they used the truck to haul dirt and other materials to construction sites, and thus was born Magliato Brothers Construction, which my brother David runs to this very day.

I am the second oldest of five children. Not a bad spot in the pecking order. It allows you to get lost in the shuffle. "Nancy, Nicky, Paul, David! Dinner!" my mom would yell from the top of our driveway to the neighborhood in general. See? Lost in the shuffle. The uniqueness of my brothers and sister is of particular interest to many people who meet me. They often assume that my mom or dad must be a doctor or, at the very least, that I have a sibling who is a physician. I am proud to say they are not and that they are all very successful and happy in the lives they have chosen. My older sister, Nancy, is the mother of six children and a guidance counselor at the local middle school in our hometown. Two of my three brothers also live in Highland near our mother and father. My youngest brother and terminal bachelor of the family, David, runs Magliato Brothers Construction, as I have said. My mid-dle brother, Paul, is married with two children and works for a construction company that builds hospitals. My oldest brother, Nick, lives in Bethesda with his wife and their twins.

He is the CEO of a software start-up company called Trust Digital.

A friend of mine once asked why it is that despite being raised in a similar manner, siblings often turn out so differently. I think that is the very definition of a family: a group of individuals, bound by the essence of love, who share a life together and yet maintain their unique individuality. That's what my family is and I love them for it.

At the helm of my diverse family are my mother and father, who both come from hardworking immigrant families with meager means. My mother's parents, Nana and Poppop, were from Germany, my father's from Italy. They met in the eighth grade, went out on a chaperoned date for a soda, and have been together ever since. Amazing. This year my parents are celebrating their fiftieth wedding anniversary, and boy, are we going to have a party! Being half Italian and half German gives me one hell of a temper, though. Someone once described my temper as an acetylene torch: I hit the target— I definitely hit the target—but I char everything around it as well. Thanks, Mom and Dad!

My mother was a high school graduate who chose a career as a homemaker. She was brilliant at it. My father attended Union College in Schenectady, New York. He graduated with a degree in industrial engineering and worked for IBM for twenty-seven years. They make a very sweet couple. My mom still lays out my dad's clothes in the morning, and my dad whistles while he cooks her dinner every night. I hope they live forever.

When I look back at all the hard work I endured in my early childhood, I realize that it had a profound impact on me as a physician. I am never daunted by hard work, whether that be long mind-numbing hours in the library during medical school, standing in the operating room as a third-year medical student gripping a retractor to hold an abdominal cavity open for a surgeon until I lost all feeling in my hands, or staying completely and utterly focused as the lead surgeon of a seventeen-hour artificial heart implant case. My dad used to say, "Hard work pays off and builds character." To that I add, "Hard work saves lives," because if you don't like to work hard, you'd best not be a surgeon.

To get away from the never-ending chores of our farm, I begged my dad to let me get a work permit when I was sixteen. That is not to say, however, that I hadn't been working for our family business since I could walk, permit or not. My first paying job was working in the outdoor maintenance crew on the Mid-Hudson Bridge. I was one of those people dressed in an orange jumpsuit swinging a Weedwacker. I am certain I was mistaken for a convict. It was grueling work in the humid summer heat of New York, and my arms, shaking with fatigue, would hang limp at my sides when my shift was over. There was very little breeze and very little rest. The only break I received was when I was allowed to paint out the rust spots on the bridge. Then I could look out over the entire Hudson valley, marvel at its beauty, and take in the cool current of air from the rolling river.

My next job was far less demanding but no less monotonous. I worked in a greenhouse and transferred sapling plants from a large holding pallet into individual smaller containers. I worked for hours on end with eyes half closed in an assembly-line setting that paid minimum wage.

The job that was responsible for changing the course of my life, however, was the job I took as a janitor at the local nursing home. I worked the night shift after school and on weekends. I did everything from scrubbing toilets to buffing floors. I took pride in my work and my evaluations consistently singled out my meticulousness, a trait that runs deep in a cardiac surgeon and one that comes naturally to me. As a potential patient, I hope you find it reassuring that the work I do inside your chest must meet my standard of perfection. If you walk into a cardiac surgeon's office and find it in complete disarray, be a little worried.

This particular nursing home had three floors. The first floor was reserved for the sickest residents, who required skilled nursing care, while the upper floors were for the more independent residents. I always asked to be assigned to the first floor because although it required more work, it allowed me to interact with the nursing staff. Occasionally a resident would become so sick that a doctor would have to make a visit to the facility. When that occurred, I would make sure that I was cleaning the sickly resident's room so that I could watch what the doctor did. I was fascinated by the contrasts. The white coat. The black bag. The grim nature of the doctor. The pleasantries of the nurse. Since all of the doctors who visited the nursing home were men, I assumed that women couldn't be doctors. That is, until my new boss arrived. Her name was Pat and she was beautiful. She had long red polished nails, drove a shiny red sports car, and wore real girl clothes, not carpenter pants that her mother bought at the hardware store in town. She was a women *and* a boss. And she was tough. White-glove-inspection tough.

So I got this idea in my sixteen-year-old head that if women could be bosses and figures of authority, then maybe women could be doctors. I wrestled with this notion for a while before I had the courage to tell anyone about it. After all, my mother wasn't a doctor and we had never had a doctor on either side of my family. I had no foundation for my own ideas about the medical world, and *Marcus Welby, M.D.* was on TV, which didn't help.

When I finally told my mother that I wanted to become a doctor, she responded by stitching a needlepoint picture of a child sitting on a fence with the caption "Your parents give you two things: One is roots and the other is wings." It was the endless encouragement of my parents, who said that I could do anything I wanted with my life, that gave me the support I needed to become a doctor. Yes, they gave me wings. Big, beautiful white wings.

I attended our local public school for elementary, middle, and high school and when I graduated from Highland High School (which surprised me, by the way, since I had toilet-papered the school, started a food fight, and burned "Class of '81" in the school's front lawn—all in my senior year), I was one of only a handful of students who went on to college. My father took me to the campus of his alma mater, Union College, and said, "Do you see this? This is what you can achieve." I was impressed with Union. My sister, my father, and his brother had all graduated from Union, so Union ran in my veins. It was a small, profoundly beautiful, private liberal arts and engineering–based curriculum school with a strong premed program. Coming from such a small town, it felt expansive. I spent four years there as a premedical undergraduate majoring in biochemistry. Despite nearly failing out in my first two trimesters, I managed to graduate with cum laude honors. Whereas high school had come easily to me, college was all about hard work and rigorous study. It just took me a while to stop partying and figure that out for myself.

During my last two years at Union College, I engaged in

an honors research project that studied the effects of a plant-derived hormone on rats. The project required me to perform surgery on the brains of rats. This was my first foray into surgery and I loved it. Instantly. Surgery and I were like two peas in a pod. We were meant to be. With surgery, you cause change almost immediately. Find a problem, fix a problem. Unlike the medical world, in which you administer a drug and wait for the result, the surgical world is about seeing the consequences of your actions the instant the scalpel is laid upon the skin, the moment a suture is passed through an artery, the second a hemostat grasps the tissue. There is a saying in surgery: "The chance to cut is the chance to cure." It is an expression suggesting that surgery cures disease while medicine simply buys you more time. For some patients, more time is enough, but not for surgeons. We want to cure. All day. Every day. Until we rid the world of disease. And so I became enamored with surgery, intoxicated by it. Caught up in the revelation that I could become this vehicle of precision and change.

I spent a term abroad in Florence, Italy, during my third year at Union. This turned out to be one of the best decisions of my life. It changed me in a way that nothing else that I had done up to that point had. I studied Renaissance art, the Italian language, and government. I got my head out of my science books for a few months and saw the world. The real, vast world with all its richness and beauty. Being in Florence, the epicenter of the Renaissance art movement, gave me an appreciation of the amazing art that can be wrought with two simple tools—the human eye and the human hand. Just stand in front of a Botticelli for five minutes and you cannot help but be inspired. Surgery is an art that inspires me. It is also an art that can save lives and change the world one person at a time. Gandhi said it best: Be the change you see in the world.

Now, before you get the idea that I am the picture of success, I must tell you a secret. A secret of which I am ashamed. A secret that bothers me to this day. *I did not get into medical school the first time that I applied.* There. I said it. Now the whole world knows and I can finally let it go. I paid the price for the lack of clarity and focus during my first two years at Union. And although when I returned from Italy, I burned through the remaining two years of college with straight A's, my grades weren't good enough.

When I sat for my prerequisite entrance exam for medical school, the MCAT, my grade on the test was less than spectacular and so—as painful as that was—I took the exam a second time. But if that was what it took to get into medical school, then that is what I did. Frankly, I would have sold my soul. In the meantime, I spent a year in a primate research laboratory performing neurosurgical procedures on monkeys and reapplied the following year. It was a year for me to hone my skills in surgery and fall deeper in love with a knife. There was just no way I was going to give up on my dream of becoming a doctor. Maybe not getting in the first time was a good thing. It certainly strengthened my resolve and commitment: I wanted medical school more than anything else in my life.

I did get into medical school that following year at Albany Medical Center in Albany, New York, and then did my final two clinical years at Case Western Reserve University School of Medicine in Cleveland, Ohio. Was it hard? You bet. Did it seem insurmountable? Absolutely. Did you ever feel like quitting? Every day. It was my passion and my parents that saw me through those long, dark hours spent in the library.

The fear of seeing your grades posted. The constant pressure of the competition among the students, so fierce at times that you never let your books out of your sight for fear that they would "go missing." We lived and died by the bell curve. I will never forget the first day of class, sitting in the lecture hall, when one of the faculty leaders walked in, and said, "Look around the room. One third of you won't be here by the end of this semester." Cutthroats, or "throats" as we called them, students who were gunning for the best grades, would see to that. And you wonder why doctors are not always compassionate. Because compassion wasn't on the bell curve.

Throughout medical school there was an ongoing discussion regarding which path you were taking—were you going to be a medical doctor or a surgeon? Like the Frost poem that describes two roads that diverge in a wood, medicine was to the right, surgery to the left. And nothing in between. I was hellbent on surgery, and so, for me, it was as if someone had put up a barricade studded with landmines across the medicine road. Yes, I took the road less traveled and, for me, it has made all the difference.

The truth is, I was bored with all of the medicine rotations that I was forced to do as a medical student—pediatrics, general inpatient medicine, outpatient medicine, psychiatry. I lived for the surgical rotations—general surgery, trauma, vascular surgery. Regardless of how I felt about the rotation, though, I was committed to learning everything, down to the most minute detail. I became a machine of instant recall. I would memorize the name and pathology of every disease, its physical findings and presentation. The workup that was needed to diagnose the problem. The treatment options. I memorized my patient's history, physical exam findings, and daily laboratory results so that at a moment's notice I could recite any of these minutiae while holding the gaze of my chief resident or attending without flinching or using a cheat sheet. For fun, I would memorize all of my patients' ten-digit medical record numbers.

The most important piece of knowledge that I learned as a medical student on the hospital wards came from the chief resident during my inpatient medical rotation at Metro County Hospital in Cleveland. As we gathered outside a cancer patient's room one day, he turned to us, the medical students, and said, "If you treat all of your patients like they are your family, you will always do right by the patient." In other words, you will always treat patients with dignity and respect. You will always spend time with your patients and check on them often. You will double- and triple-check the patient's tests and laboratories. You will follow up on every result. You will show compassion. You will hold your patient's hand as she lies on the operating table and slowly drifts toward a deep sleep under anesthesia. You will wipe away her tears when she is in pain and frustrated at not being able to communicate with you because she is stuck on a ventilator. You will hug her good-bye when she asks you "How can I thank you, doctor?" on her way out the door upon discharge. I have repeated this same teaching "to treat patients like family" to the many medical students, residents, and nurses whom I've taught throughout the years. It is, in my opinion, the surest way to live up to the Hippocratic oath.

4

The Hand of a Lady

A SURGEON IN TRAINING

BELIEVE THAT I FARE BETTER AS A BIGGER FISH IN A smaller pond rather than a smaller fish in a bigger pond, so when it came time for me to emerge from the sheltered cocoon of postgraduate education and morph into a doctor in clinical training, I chose a residency program at a small hospital in Akron, Ohio, called Akron General Medical Center. I had entertained general surgery residency positions at large university programs, but in the end Akron just felt right. And surgeons are all about gut instincts. I spent a total of six years in my general surgery residency: the first year as an intern, year two as a junior resident, year three in a research fellowship at the University of Michigan Medical Center, years four and five back at Akron as a senior resident, and year six as a chief resident. It was 1990 and I was the first woman ever to be accepted into the surgery program there—a pattern that I would see over and over again in my training. There just weren't many women surgeons at that time. Sadly, women still remain a minority in surgery.

My general surgery training molded me as a surgeon. It challenged the core of who I was a surgeon and as a human being. But it also did something to me that wasn't so gallant. It made me build what I call my full-metal jacket. Being the first woman in the program was difficult, to say the least. I was constantly challenged to see "just how much she could take." One of the rites of passage as a general surgeon usually occurs while on the trauma rotation. It is a procedure called an ER thoracotomy, which is done to patients who have experienced a traumatic event so severe that it has caused them to arrest. Gunshot wounds, stab wounds, and high-impact motor vehicle accidents are examples of such events. An ER thoracotomy is done in the emergency room and involves rapidly opening the side of the chest, identifying and clamping the aorta, and opening the sac around the heart to relieve a buildup of blood and to perform open heart massage. The goal is to restore blood pressure and keep patients alive to transport them to an operating room for definitive treatment. I overheard my male counterparts talking about me one day, saying that they felt I would not be able to perform an ER thoracotomy when the time came, that I would simply "chicken out." Lo and behold, my time did come during my third year of residency, and when called upon to perform an ER thoracotomy on a dying trauma victim, I sliced him open like a ripe melon, reached into his chest and fished around in what felt like pumpkin guts to find the aorta, clamped it, and brought back the patient's blood pressure. It took a certain amount of what surgeons like to call testicular fortitude to do this, but it also helped to have a full-metal jacket.

My full-metal jacket was unique to me. It fit me perfectly because I had constructed it inch by inch. Tailored, if you will, to conform to my exact shape. Made of mithril, when I wore it, I was impervious to pain. My pain. My patient's pain. The pain of the world around me. I could take on any challenge without fear of being harmed—I felt nothing. Emotionally, spiritually, psychologically. It made me so tough. It allowed me to survive. The problem was that when I wore this jacket, no one could get close to me. Not my colleagues. Not my patients. It was as if I had a force field around me, and I liked it that way. The jacket was somewhat versatile. I could wear it on the outside of my clothing for all to see my virility or wear it on the inside so I just exuded toughness. The trade-off was that when I wore it, I couldn't be a woman. I couldn't look like a woman. I couldn't act like a woman. Because weren't women weak? They certainly weren't surgeons.

When I look back on it now, I realize that I wore that jacket every day for a long, long time—indeed, throughout all of my training as a surgeon. And sometimes, it was the only thing holding me together . . .

• • •

I didn't know the patient at all. Never met her before or after the surgery. I was detached. *Detached*, because I was a "rotator" on the orthopedic service. I was not part of the core team but merely a spectator on the periphery. When you are an intern, you rotate (hence the label rotator) through a multitude of surgical subspecialties. Like some rude game of spin the bottle, you briefly kiss each specialty—vascular surgery, plastic surgery, orthopedic surgery, neurosurgery—but never follow through on the promise of that interaction. Never commit to any long-term relationship. *Detached*, because I was a nonexistent entity in the OR that day and was told to "show up, shut up and wear beige." In other words, "Just melt into the background, lowly intern, and don't touch anything."

We were doing a forequarter resection that awful day on a woman who had an upper-arm malignant sarcoma invading into her shoulder. Sarcomas are particularly nasty cancers, which, when they occur in an extremity, usually require an amputation as treatment. At least they did eighteen years ago when I was an intern.

In this patient's case, we were going to take her arm clean off, including the shoulder joint. I am dead serious. Dead and buried serious. We were going to literally *detach* (there's that word again) this woman's entire upper extremity, very matter-of-factly, from the rest of her body. When the orthopedic surgeon told me what we were about to do, he made it sound like it was some routine, easy-as-pie operation, as if the patient were a Mrs. Potato Head and we were just changing out her arm for one with a tennis racket in it. I was horrified. I was disgusted. I could barely swallow my own spit. But like an obedient intern, I showed up, shut my mouth, wore beige, and blended in like a chameleon on a rock, hoping they didn't need me.

They did.

"*Hold* the arm and *pull*," I was told. Not *her* arm. *The* arm. Somehow, by not using the female pronoun, it allowed me to have just a modicum of distance from the operation. *Hold, pull.* Two simple commands, but you have no idea how difficult it was to actually do it.

So there I stood, wordlessly holding this poor woman's arm the way a fireman holds on to a fire hose under the pressure of a full gust of water. I tucked her biceps under my

armpit and held a firm grip with my right hand on her elbow
and my left hand on her wrist. I leaned away from her using
my weight to pull *the* arm (not *her* arm) from its socket. In this
manner, I kept my back to her for the entire operation as if by
putting the procedure behind me, literally, I was somehow less
involved.

And if that weren't bad enough, the worst part was that
as I held the arm in my viselike grip, I could feel everything
the surgeons were doing to detach it. Like putting your ear to
a train track and feeling the vibration of an oncoming loco-
motive, I could feel the coarse, scratching movements as they
cut the gristle of each ligament and tendon. The vibrations
traveled from her shoulder down her arm to where I gripped
it at the forearm and wrist. That's when I suddenly and fully
mentally *detached* from the operation. From the patient. Like
pulling the rip cord on a parachute or dropping your weight
belt while scuba diving, I just needed to float away from what
was happening. *Right. Now.*

I did this by running the periodic table of elements in my
head. The periodic table of elements is a tabular form dis-
playing all of the known chemical elements in existence. Formulated in 1869, there are, as of January 2008, 117 elements.
As a biochemistry major, the most extreme form of mental tor-
ture that I had to endure was to memorize the entire table,
which included knowing the names of all of the elements as
well as their atomic number (number of protons in their nu-
cleus), quantum electron configuration, and their state of matter at standard temperature and pressure (0 degrees C and one
standard atmosphere). My favorite group of chemical elements, should you want to know, was the last column of the
table, which housed the noble gases. Not only did I like the

name *noble gases*, but I also liked the fact that these gases were chemically inert because they were extremely stable. These gases have a full valence shell of electrons, which is the holy grail of all chemical elements because they don't need to react with any other elements in the table to scavenge electrons. I further liked the fact that krypton was one of the noble gases. The Superman of the periodic table.

Such were my musings while we took this patient's arm off. The periodic table of elements distracted me from what was going on and kept me mentally detached from my gruesome surroundings. That was until the surgeons finally (and mercifully) cut the last attachments. I lurched forward a few steps because I had my weight shifted away from the patient. This jarred me from my helium-neon-argon-krypton-xenon-radon reverie. We were detached, the arm and I. We were free. Free to be discarded. Free to exhale.

I stood there blinking with amazement until the realization that I was holding a human limb in my arms slowly, yet vividly, began to sink in. No one acknowledged me. At all. No one cared. No one told me what to do with the arm. No one cared. They no longer cared about the arm, *her* arm. They no longer cared about me. We had both become useless appendages.

The surgeons were busy examining the remaining bloody stump, trying to identify the cut ends of muscle and sinew. Their job was to figure out how to tuck them all back in again and make a neat a package of it. So I stood there, like an idiot, holding the arm. An arm that once could gesture beautifully like that of a prima ballerina, if it wished, and raise itself gracefully against gravity. The arm was heavy now, a victim of gravity because it could no longer move against it. I held my breath. I held the arm. I waited to be told what to do next. The arm grew heavy. Time slowed to an agonizing halt.

That's when I really got the hell out of there and detached from the scene. I went to Normandy. In my mind, I pictured myself at the landing on Omaha Beach during World War II. I was a medic whose job it was to gather all of the dismembered limbs from the injured soldiers and make a pile. *Gather. Pile.* Again, two simple commands. I could do this, I thought to myself, I am a medic in World War II and this is my job. My duty to my fellow soldiers. My honor for their honor. I could do this.

I snapped out of my battlefield delusion when I heard the orthopedic surgeon finally say, "Put it over there," and gesture to a large plastic specimen bin. I cradled the arm and gently, almost lovingly, deposited it in the tray as if it were my own child whom I was putting down for an afternoon nap in his crib.

If it had not been for the shielding that was provided to me by my full-metal jacket that day, I'm afraid I would have come undone. A fragmented mess. A splintered pile of black and blue broken tile. Worthless rubbish. Useless to everyone in the OR including the patient. But wearing that protective gear sheltered me from feeling anything about this dismembered woman. It was a trade-off that, at the time, I had to make for my own self-preservation.

Many years have passed since my intern days, and yet I still feel such remorse for having detached myself from the operation and, ultimately, the patient that I never did it again. No matter how gruesome an operation can get. This was possibly one of the most important events in this woman's life. One that would change her forever. I am mortified that I stood like a stone in the OR and never imagined the impact this would have on her, so preoccupied was I about the impact it would have on me. I feel absolutely awful that I never wondered anything about this woman. I never wondered, for example, how she felt about losing her arm. I never wondered if she stood in the mirror the evening before the surgery and moved slowly to the left until her arm disappeared from the reflection. Did she do this to imagine how she would look without her arm? I never wondered if she would miss the symmetry of her upper body. Did she kneel and pray that night for a safe operation with both hands, fingertips touching piously in their final clasp? Did she hug her children good-bye the following morning, the day of the operation, with the last two-armed embrace they will ever know? Did she bow her head for the last time and cry into the comfort of both cupped hands as she was driven to the hospital? I never wondered any of this, for how can a stone, a stone wearing a full-metal jacket, wonder?

No. Never again. When I operate, I am fully aware of who is beneath my drapes, what I am doing to them, and how it will affect their lives forever. I keep my head *and* my heart in the game. I remain, at all times, solemnly, devotedly, attached.

But I survived it. The tearing off of a limb. I survived that and so much more . . .

• • •

As a general surgery resident, at a time when I was searching my soul for some kind of justification for what I was having to endure each day, Dr. Kayman, the most senior staff surgeon, said the most amazing thing to me. One day, during an inguinal hernia repair, he touched my hand and said, "In order to be not just a good surgeon but a great surgeon, you need the eye of an eagle, the heart of a lion, and the hand of a lady." When he said it he had the most amazing twinkle in his eye, like my grandfather's, and despite his surgical mask, I could see him smiling proudly at me. And I thought, "My God, maybe I could be a surgeon."

If general surgery was so tough, why pursue a career in the biggest boys' club of them all, cardiac surgery? Two words: *the heart.* I was pursuing the heart itself as much as I was pursuing a career because I was so enamored with it as a life-sustaining entity. My husband (a liver transplant surgeon) and I are in a constant debate about which organ is the most important—the heart or the liver. But seriously, folks, how can you respect an organ you can eat?

And so, with my newfound fondness and commitment to the heart, I applied to many cardiothoracic training programs around the United States during my fourth year as a general surgery resident. The competition for training spots was fierce. Whenever I went for an interview, I was always the only woman who had applied for that program. I was always asked the same question: "You're a woman. Why would you want to be a heart surgeon?" The interviewer would always have that same incredulous look on his face. I couldn't tell him about the first time I touched the heart because that was too "girly" an answer. So I just came up with some canned answer that seemed to placate the interviewer. What I really wanted to say was, "Do you ask the guys this same question?" but I knew to keep my mouth shut.

Once, during an interview, I was asked, "What happens if you get pregnant during your training?" I thought about it for a minute and answered confidently, "I guess I'd just stand farther from the operating table" (which, by the way, is exactly what I did when I was pregnant and operating). Needless to say, I didn't get into *that* program. At one very prestigious university, I was asked to meet for my interview with a cardiothoracic surgeon in the OR instead of his office. I was given a locker key and directed to the OR locker room, where I was to change into surgical scrubs and go to the surgeon's operating room. Just as I had stripped down to my bra and underwear, I heard what distinctly sounded like a man urinating in a toilet. To my utter surprise, I heard the toilet flush, and out of the adjoining bathroom walked a man in scrubs. I stood there in what can only be described as a classic Maidenform moment advertisement. Nice. He looked me up down and said, "What are you doing in here?" I was so flustered that I couldn't think of anything to say except "I'm interviewing for a residency position." He smirked at me and said in a lascivious tone, "I'll just bet you are, little girl." When I confronted the residency program director about the fact that I had been directed to the male locker room instead of the female locker room, he laughed and said that because no other women had applied to the program, he had sent me to the male locker room out of habit. Honest mistake? Or was he just trying to ensure that I wouldn't consider their hospital's training program? Either way, I didn't rank that program among those I wanted to attend. No harm. No foul.

Despite the grueling interview process, I did manage to procure one of the coveted spots in a cardiothoracic surgery training program in Chicago and began what were the most taxing two years of my life. The residency was made all the more difficult by the fact that, again, I was the only woman to go through the program. I shared an on-call room, bathroom, and shower with three male residents. After a while, it was just like sharing the single bathroom we had in my house growing up with my three brothers. I borrowed their toothpaste, they borrowed my shampoo. I got used to their snoring, they got used to my stealing all the covers. Together and apart, we made it through those two years. We loved each other, hated each other, covered for each other, and ratted each other out.

On more than one occasion, I was so sleep deprived that I actually started dreaming while awake and couldn't differentiate dream from reality. I lost weight. I lost interest. I lost contact with my friends, the world at large, and even my family. I wrapped my full-metal jacket around me for warmth and protection and somehow faced each day. We had a running contest to see who could spend the most consecutive days in the hospital without leaving to go home. My record was eleven days before I was later disqualified for leaving the hospital to buy a clean pair of underwear. When I finally finished the program, I was given a gift from one my residency "brothers." It was a pocket-size version of *The Art of War* by Sun Tzu. On the inside front cover he wrote, "Thanks for watching my back. I hope this book comes in handy as you do battle during the coming years. Take no prisoners." On the back cover he wrote, "The surest way to defeat an enemy is to make him your sincerest friend." I still keep it in the pocket of my white coat and take it out from time to time to remind me of the most difficult passage of my life.

It was 1998 when I finished my training as a cardiothoracic surgeon, and instead of taking the sane path of finding a job as a full-fledged heart surgeon (known as an attending surgeon), I again took the road less traveled and opted to do another fellowship training year in heart transplantation. Why? you ask. Because even more fun than touching the human heart each day is cutting out the human heart from the chest and holding it up in your hand to behold. That is a privilege that very few heart surgeons get to have. In fact, only heart transplant surgeons have the opportunity to experience this amazing feat and I wanted to be one of them. I already had been training for eight years since graduating from medical school. What's another year? Really.

I entered the heart/lung transplant fellowship program at the University of Pittsburgh Medical Center, one of the most well-respected and prestigious transplant training programs in the country. I felt proud to be a part of this team. For the next year I would learn about the art of transplantation. From the nuances of how to surgically perform the transplant proce-dures to how these difficult patients are managed medically after they receive their donor heart or lung. I learned how to manipulate one of the most complex and poorly understood systems in the human body—the immune system. We used powerful drugs to suppress the immune system that caused patients to "shake and bake," as we called it, which meant they developed high fevers and seizures while being administered the medications. It was a tightrope of daily micromanaging the amounts of the drug that were delivered—too much of the drugs and they develop an infection or cancer that would kill them, too little of the drugs and they die of organ rejection. I found it all fascinating.

When I arrived at the University of Pittsburgh in July of 1998, my first task was to learn how to extract the heart and lungs from a donor and preserve them in such a way as to keep them viable for transport back to Pittsburgh in working condition. Because the human heart cannot be out of one body for more than four hours before being implanted into another, it was no easy feat to recover donor organs. The process of retrieving a donor organ at a distant medical center went like this: We had to be transported by ambulance to a heliport station in Pittsburgh to be flown by helicopter to a local airfield, where we picked up a private jet that would take us to a private airport nearest to the hospital where the donor was being prepped for surgery. We were then transported by ambulance or helicopter from the airfield to the donor's hospital. In the OR were several teams of surgeons, each retrieving the particular organ that was designated for the recipient back at their own hospital—liver, two kidneys, pancreas, small intestine, two eyes, skin, bones, two lungs, heart. One generous donor can save so many lives. The heart team is the lead team during a procurement, because the heart is taken out first, followed by the remainder of the organs. When the aorta is clamped, blocking all flow from the heart, the heart is freed from its attachments in the chest and removed. The patient then moves from a state of brain death to a pulseless, complete death. This transition to death, a transition that I was directly responsible for, was always a profound moment for me personally. A very solemn, profound moment during which I always prayed for the donor and the family and quietly thanked them for their ultimate gift—the gift of life for someone whom they will never know.

Once the aorta is clamped, the clock begins to tick, and the race begins. We now have to get the heart out of the chest, preserve and package it for the long transport back to Pittsburgh, and then take the ambulance–helicopter–jet–helicopter–ambulance transport system to our hospital. We may be as far away as Florida or Texas and still have to do this *and* sew the heart into the recipient in under four hours! Incredible. It was a year of extreme fatigue and adrenaline rushes all intertwined into a helix that became my DNA. It was a year of saving lives. A year of taking the most horrible of situations—the tragic death of a loved one—and spinning it into the most rewarding gift of life for the recipient. For me the year was bipolar, with highs being very high and the lows being so low I thought they would crush me, full-metal jacket and all.

The first donor run, as we called it, that I participated in occurred a mere two days after setting foot inside the University of Pittsburgh Medical Center. It was the middle of the night and I was told to show up at the emergency room entrance in ten minutes to catch an ambulance to the airport, where a plane awaited to take me to one of the largest and most prestigious university hospitals in the Midwest. This middle-of-the-night donor run seemed like a welcome relief because I was at that time sleeping on the floor of my apartment with nothing but a pillow and a sky-blue afghan that my nana had knit me, since my furniture had not yet arrived from Chicago. Sleeping in a private plane sounded like heaven. When I arrived at the emergency room ambulance dock, I was told we would be taking the donor heart from a three-day-old infant who had sustained a head-crush injury during a difficult delivery with a forceps. I hadn't the faintest idea how to procure a pediatric donor heart or any donor heart for that matter. Thankfully, Mike, a senior resident in cardiothoracic surgery, was going to accompany me on the trip and he had done the procedure before. I was so nervous about the surgery that I didn't sleep at all on the plane and he and I spent the trip rehearsing how we were going to remove this little angel's heart.

When we arrived at the university hospital, the chief of the Cardiothoracic Surgery Department himself greeted us in the OR and thought he would watch "just to make sure everything goes smoothly." As if I weren't under enough pressure. We entered the OR suite to find, to my dismay, that the baby wasn't yet draped on the operating table. This forced me to have to look at this most beautiful donor before I split its chest open and set it free. As pristine as this baby was on the outside, it was just as pristine on the inside because, unlike an adult, a baby's heart is free of any fat or scar that might mar its surface. We painstakingly removed the heart with such delicate surgical moves so as not to injure the precious gift, since it is rare to get a pediatric heart transplant from such a young donor. For a fleeting moment I was able to hold that little bird heart, no larger than a silver dollar, in the palm of my hand. Not for a long time, though, because my body heat would warm it in my hand and destroy the preservation that is sustained through cooling with ice and iced solutions. Warm hands, cold heart. I carried that cold little heart, cupped in my warm hands, to the transport cooler as if it were the Hope diamond itself because to me, there is nothing so precious as the heart of a donor child.

For weeks after we implanted the heart into the recipient baby, I struggled with the knowledge that I had taken that donor baby's heart and allowed it to pass through death's door. When I heard that the recipient baby had done well and was ready for discharge, I went to the baby's room where the parents were swaddling their infant, preparing for home. I told the parents who I was and what I had done. I told them that I had been struggling with the task that I had needed to perform in order to save their baby's life. They smiled at me—actually smiled. I guess I thought they would see me as some kind of grave-robbing Frankenstein. I was wrong. Then they asked me if I wanted to hold their baby and I said yes. I took that little child in my arms and cradled him with one hand while putting my other hand on his chest to feel the heartbeat. The heartbeat was strong. It was persistent. Life is persistent, love is persistent, and yes, the heart is persistent.

Three hundred sixty-four long days and longer nights later, I graduated from the transplant program at Pittsburgh. Donor and recipient. Death and life. Yin and yang. It was indeed a year of extremes and I had survived. I could now sit for my board exams and finally look for a job. A real job. With my first real paycheck. I was thirty-six years old.

5

Drop-dead Gorgeous

THERE ARE THOSE PEOPLE FOR WHOM OPPORTUNITY always seems to knock. Not me. I have never waited for opportunity to find me, I have always ventured out in search of it.

• • •

As an intern in general surgery, you were constantly under the watchful eye of the more senior residents, especially when you were doing a procedure on a patient. Even if I was removing a mere skin tag on a patient's arm, I would have a senior resident looking over my shoulder.

RESIDENT: Cut there.

ME: Where? Here, right in front of me where this big, obvious-as-the-nose-on-your-face skin tag is?

RESIDENT: Yes. And don't press too hard on the scalpel and cut too deep.

ME: Oh, so you don't want me to cut all the way to the bone?

RESIDENT: No. It's just the little floppy piece of skin that we're cutting off.

ME: So we're not taking off the whole arm below the elbow?

RESIDENT: No. Just the skin tag.

And so it went. The resident speaking to me as if I were a blind two-year-old and me, the defiant two-year-old, fighting for a little independence. Just a modicum of autonomy. Hey, I was already toilet trained . . .

RESIDENT: Put one stitch right here.

ME: Not fifty-seven?

RESIDENT: No. Just one.

ME: Where? On the forehead?

RESIDENT: No. Where you made your incision . . .

After months and months of tutelage your first chance to "fly solo" as an intern came when you had to put in a Greenfield filter. It was the simplest of procedures (simpler than a skin tag removal), but the cool thing was, you got to do the procedure in an OR. *Your* OR. With your very own nurse and everything!

A Greenfield filter looks like a badminton birdie. It is placed in a large vein called the vena cava. The filter acts like a catcher's mitt and will catch and cage any large deep venous thrombosis in your leg and prevent it from traveling to the right side of your heart and out into the pulmonary artery to cause a fatal pulmonary embolism.

I loved doing Greenfield filters because they satisfied my need for autonomy and independent decision making. I decided, after inserting a few filters successfully, that I would track down Dr. Lazar J. Greenfield, inventor of the Greenfield filter, and thank him personally for making a device so simple that even an intern could implant it. He was, at that time, the chairman of the Department of Surgery at the University of Michigan Medical Center. He was a big fish in a big pond and I saw an opportunity . . .

The first chance I got, I drove from Ohio to Michigan, completely unannounced. I located his office, slipped past his secretary, and just knocked on his door.

"Hi!" I said, trying not to look or sound like a stalker. "I'm Kathy Magliato, a general surgery intern from Ohio, and I just wanted to thank you—"

"How'd you get here?" He seemed a little perplexed.

"I drove."

"You drove all the way from Ohio just to thank me for inventing the Greenfield filter?" he said, looking at me as if I *were* a stalker.

"Yes."

Dr. Greenfield was so impressed that he took me around the hospital with him and introduced me to the general surgery attending surgeons in his department. By the end of the day, they asked me if I would like to come back and spend a few months on the transplant service learning liver and kidney transplantation. Since we did not have a transplant program at my hospital, this was quite the opportunity indeed.

And so I returned the following year to spend a rotation on the transplant service at the University of Michigan Medical Center. It was a magical few months of surgery I might otherwise never have seen. A nonstop parade of livers and kidneys and pancreases (oh my!), livers and kidneys and pancreases (oh my!). And although the first liver transplant was done in 1963, the first successful kidney transplant was in 1954, and the first pancreas transplant was in 1966, it all felt brand-new to me. I guess I was just a wide-eyed junior resident caught up in the romance of transplantation.

The transplant service was, by far, the busiest of all the surgical services. We were either putting organs in, changing them out for new ones when they didn't work right away, or taking patients back to the OR when they leaked from arteries, veins, ureters, bile ducts—anything that was sewn together between donor organ and recipient. They should have had a revolving door on our OR, *that's* how busy we were.

Michigan is where I did my first transplant and for that I am eternally grateful. It was a kidney transplant in a young man. The donor was a tragedy—a gorgeous young woman who simply dropped dead from sudden cardiac arrest. This blew my mind because I had never experienced a case of sudden cardiac death. Young, healthy, and in her early thirties, she just fell over dead in her tracks one day. Sudden cardiac arrest is so alarming because it is a swift execution by the heart that occurs without warning. In fact, it is the leading cause of natural death, killing 450,000 people each year. Ninety-five percent of people who experience sudden cardiac arrest die. The other 5 percent are nothing short of a miracle. It is a merciless killer in that it is commonly seen in young adults in their thirties and forties who appear healthy and have no heart disease.

Sudden cardiac death is an electrical malfunction of the heart that flips the heartbeat into a fast, irregular rhythm know as ventricular fibrillation. Ventricular fibrillation causes the lower chambers of the heart to quiver instead of beat and no blood is pumped to the body. Most people think that sudden cardiac death is the same as a heart attack. It is not, although it can occur during a heart attack, as was the case with Tim Russert. According to published reports, Russert was in a sound studio at the Washington, D.C., bureau of NBC news recording voice-overs for *Meet the Press*. At approximately 1:30 p.m. on June 13, 2008, he suddenly collapsed without warning. Co-workers administered mouth-to-mouth resuscitation and called 911. Emergency Medical Services were called at 1:40 p.m. and arrived at 1:44 p.m. They found Russert in ventricular fibrillation and shocked him three times without success. He was pronounced dead at a local hospital at 2:23 p.m. His autopsy showed that a large plaque in the main artery that courses down the front of the heart had ruptured, cutting off blood supply to a large portion of the heart and causing it to fibrillate.

Automatic external defibrillators (AEDs) are available in most public places and can be used by the layperson to shock someone who has had a sudden cardiac arrest. Unfortunately for Tim and for the woman who donated her kidney, an AED was not available. And so this young woman, this tragedy of circumstances, opened the door to a career in transplantation for me, the greatest of gifts that she unknowingly gave.

The transplant itself was an ephemeral experience. The operation is rather short and fairly straightforward—you simply have to connect three things—the artery, the vein, and the ureter—so that arterial blood, venous blood, and urine can flow to and from the kidney, respectively. Success is measured by urine output. The happier the kidney, the more urine it makes. I wanted my first kidney transplant to last longer than the transiency of the operation, so while the patient was in the recovery room, I collected some of the urine in a bottle and carried it around with me the rest of the day on rounds. I was so proud of my vial of urine that I only let a select few of my closest colleagues have a peek at it, as if it were liquid gold.

Rounds on the transplant service were intense. We marched around in silence completely focused on the task of seeing each of the incredibly complex patients on our service. One could hear a pin drop in the hallway ahead of us and nothing but the rush of the air in our wake. Focus, focus, focus. Every detail of every patient was combed over. The intensity was made worse by "the Book." The Book was the Gideon Bible of the transplant service. It was a five ring notebook filled with pages and pages of patient data. In those days, we didn't have computers keeping track of our patients' medications and laboratory values. We did it the old-fashioned way—by scribe. When it was your turn to hold the Book, you were in charge of compiling all of the patient data for the service—their lab results, their X-ray results, their biopsy results, what medications they were on, their immunosuppression dosages and levels. It was all handwritten *in pen* in the Book. You were not allowed to use pencil, and use of Wite-Out was considered a sign of weakness. Each mark in the Book had to be perfect and it had to be correct, or you might just as well hang up your scalpel, shameful one.

The Book, incidentally, was also a running log. Each patient had one page and the data were cumulative from day to day. Lose the Book and you would lose the entire medical history of that patient's stay in the hospital. Lose the Book, lose your job. I have post-traumatic stress disorder just thinking about it. I took the Book everywhere with me. To the bathroom (in the stall with me), to the bedroom (under my pillow at night). We were inseparable. I was one with the Book and the Book was one with me.

We should all have a Book in our lives—something we cling to, something that yields knowledge, something that gives us purpose—no matter how crazy you think it is. But medicine isn't like that anymore. The young surgical residents who are coming up through the ranks don't seem to have that sense of dire responsibility. This frightens me because instilling that sense of ultimate responsibility and dedication is quite difficult to do; it really must come naturally.

I didn't just survive the transplant service at Michigan, I blossomed from it. Intense, smart, focused, I returned to Ohio ready to take on the remaining years of my surgical residency. I did so well at Michigan that they invited me to take a year off from my surgery training and spend time in a research laboratory studying lung transplantation in rats. In 1993, between my third and fourth years of general surgery training, I returned to Ann Arbor. The year that I spent in the lab was a year of respite from the grueling detail of general surgery. I bought a bicycle and leisurely biked to the hospital every day. I showered every morning and ate three meals a day. Sometimes, I even had lunch outside! Imagine that. Each day, I sewed donor lungs into recipient rats using a surgical microscope. It was difficult and tedious. One misstep, one slight tremor, and you would make an infinitesimal tear in the connecting vessel and the recipient would die right there under the scope. I killed a lot of rats, but in the process I perfected my technique and learned to be a meticulously accurate seamstress. The first rat that survived was E. You can imagine what happened to A, B, C, and D. I let him live at the conclusion of our experiments and he became the lab mascot. I took him home with me when I returned to Ohio and E lived for many years with his lung transplant. He was my inspiration for success.

You can see that in my life one opportunity builds upon another. Spotting that opportunity and taking full advantage of it is the difficult part, but it's a lesson I learned early on. And I would encourage all of you to constantly scan your life in search of where an opportunity may lie, veiled in the confusion of your daily grind. Don't wait for it to find you because it might just pass you by.

6

Boys Will Be Boys

We only see so far because we stand on the shoulders of giants.

—Isaac Newton

WHEN I WAS IN MY RESIDENCY IN CARDIOTHORACIC SUR-
gery, I would carry a book with me to any and every surgery
conference that I attended. The book is titled *Surgery of the
Chest* and is written by Dr. David C. Sabiston Jr. and Dr. Frank
C. Spencer. Although the book is coauthored, among cardiothoracic surgeons it is referred to as just "Sabiston." Not "*the*
(long *e*) Sabiston" or "Sabiston's textbook." Just "Sabiston," as
in "Did you read Sabiston, the chapter on the Belsey Mark IV
Antireflux repair?" (Incidentally, I once met Dr. Belsey and
asked him why he called it the Mark IV repair and he answered, "Because the other three didn't work." The man had a
sense of humor, no doubt.)

Dr. Sabiston is one the pioneers of cardiothoracic surgery,
having performed one of the first bypass surgeries in a human
patient in 1962. He served as the chief of Cardiothoracic Surgery at Duke University in Durham, North Carolina, for
thirty-two years, and his residency program was notorious as

one of the most difficult and grueling. He was a man to be both admired and feared. If I had been his resident, he probably would have eaten me alive.

His book is the bible of cardiothoracic surgery. Written in two volumes, it contains 2,174 pages, not including the nearly 100-page index, and if you put it on your bathroom scale (which I did), it weighs in at 15.7 pounds. The first volume of the sixth edition contains 1,099 pages and is the one that I carried with me cradled in my arms like a schoolgirl. I would attend these surgical conferences for the express purpose of seeking out the giants of cardiothoracic surgery and getting them to sign my book. Alas, some might consider this stalking. But these living legends of cardiothoracic surgery were superstars to me—the Julius Ervings of heart surgery—and the only place where I would ever have the opportunity to come into contact with them was at a national surgery convention. If you want to meet a rock star, you go to a rock concert, right?

I was very bold in my pursuit of their signatures. I would literally just walk right up to the particular legend whom I had in my sights, push away the throngs of wannabes and picture takers who surrounded him, and simply say, "Excuse me, I'm Kathy Magliato, a cardiothoracic resident in training. Would you sign my Sabiston?" They would always smile at me with a look of intrigue and were very gracious about signing. I think they humored me because I was a chick. When I attempted to get the signature of Christiaan Barnard, the surgeon credited with performing the first heart transplant and one of my most coveted signatures to date, he said, "Why don't we go somewhere private and I'll sign your book." He must have been at least thirty years my senior, but you can't fault the guy for trying. Besides, I already knew about his reputation for enjoying the company of young women and was prepared for this. "That would be great," I said, "but it's gonna be awfully hard for you to operate with broken fingers." He pondered this for a minute as if actually weighing broken fingers against the potential sexual conquest and said, "I like your spirit. Will you at least join me at my table for lunch?" and just like that, I got to have lunch with a rock star.

His table was filled with a *Who's Who* of heart surgery. I spent the lunch wide-eyed, completely engrossed in the conversation without eating a thing. Everyone around the table was telling stories about heart surgery and reminiscing. I am certain the majority of the surgeons at the table thought that I was Christiaan Barnard's latest lover. Sorry to disappoint, but Dr. Barnard was the perfect gentleman and I, the perfect lady. After lunch he signed my book and the inscription read:

> *To Kathy,*
> *with lots of love*
> *Christiaan Barnard*

While this may seem like an inappropriate inscription in a surgical textbook, to me it perfectly reflects the spirit of Barnard.

My first mentor in cardiothoracic surgery was Dr. Lars Vista. Like Barnard, he was a character in his own right. He was gruff and moody and swore like a truck driver. Anyone who crossed him, or whom he didn't think highly of, he referred to as a rat-fucker. As in, "Did you see what that rat-fucker did to my patient?"—referring to a consultant who had, perhaps, intervened in the patient's care. You couldn't really engage him in conversation because apart from the cursing he didn't talk much. His answers were always curt and he barked simple orders such as "Fix that" when a patient's heart rate dropped to a dangerous level or "Tap that" when a patient had too much fluid in his lungs. He never gave any details such as which patient or which lung to tap or which medication he wanted to use to remedy the heart rate problem. These he simply left you, the cowering resident, to figure out by osmosis.

He chain-smoked, lighting one cigarette with the next, and as a consequence had a coarse, raspy voice that sounded like he ate gravel for breakfast. How ironic that a man who is a champion of trying to wipe out heart disease was a habitual smoker. Such was his addiction that he would literally scrub out of an open heart case to sneak off to a small room adjoining his OR (away from the oxygen, thank God) to have a smoke.

The guy was tough and he was mean—my two favorite traits of his. I don't know, I guess I just liked the fact that he was a quintessential curmudgeon. Hey, at least he wasn't a wallflower like some of the other heart surgeons I had encountered in my training. He kept to himself and didn't cavort with other doctors. He was the master of his own universe and marched to the beat of his own drum. He didn't care what others thought of him. As surgery residents we learned to steer clear of him and adhere to the "don't speak unless spoken to" principle when it was absolutely necessary to be in his presence. In his eyes, we, the lowly residents, were rat-fuckers and therefore were *absolutely forbidden* to conduct rounds on or take care of his patients under penalty of death. Unless, of course, he barked an order at you to do so.

I, however, found a chink in his armor. He was a true historian of cardiothoracic surgery. Like a World War II veteran, he could recount the greatest milestones and battles in heart and lung surgery because he had been there. He had lived it. He had trained in cardiothoracic surgery from 1965 to 1975 during some of the greatest times of discovery in the field. He did residencies at the most prestigious hospitals at that time and worked with surgeons who pioneered techniques such as hypothermia (cooling patients during surgery), which led to the earliest developments of the pacemaker. Since I was such a cardiac history buff and, as you know, a devoted "groupie" of its pioneers, he and I would spend hours in his office discussing the "greatest hits" of thoracic surgery. We communicated on this one plane because we shared a love for the past. And out of this love grew the friendship between a mentor and his pupil.

Our discussions were such a thrill for me because the man spoke to no one and never allowed anyone into his private office. His inner sanctum was just what you'd expect it to look like. From floor to ceiling his office was stacked with books and medical journals. An avid reader, he would brag that he read twelve journals each month. You can tell whether or not a doctor reads his journals by their appearance. If they are neatly stacked and have pristine covers, then no, the information contained inside the journal has not made it into the doctor's brain. The journals are for decoration only. In Dr. Vista's office, the journals were strewn about with no logical filing system that I could ever discern. But if you asked him for "the *Journal of Thoracic and Cardiovascular Surgery* from May 1984, volume two, the supplement, please," he could somehow pull it out of thin air. The journals were all in disrepair—folded grotesquely in half or rolled up into a weapon of sorts with edges tattered or frankly torn. Pages worth noting had folded-back corners, or if an article really caught his eye, then the pages were ripped out from the journal's spine like some macabre dismemberment. Yes, there was no mistaking it. He had read the hell out of these scientific manuscripts.

There was absolutely no room, by the way, to sit down, and you really didn't want to because every ten minutes or so you needed to leave the room to take in a little smoke-free air. The smoky staleness of that office was incredible. You left there feeling as though you had licked an ashtray. Every inch of surface was covered in the dense brownish yellow staining of nicotine. You could wet your finger, run it along his office window, and write your name legibly. If that man didn't give me cancer, then I am truly invincible.

Our mentor-student discussions would take us on a journey through the distinct history of cardio (heart) and thoracic (lung) surgery. Inevitably, we would start by talking about the birth of lung surgery, which predates heart surgery. Lung surgery was born from the treatment of tuberculosis (TB) in the nineteenth century. At first TB was largely treated in sanatoriums where patients were isolated and treated with rest and fresh air. The medical doctors began to notice, however, that patients who developed a pneumothorax (collapsed lung) tended to fare better. They began to utilize "collapse therapy" to treat TB, thinking that by collapsing the lung it could rest and heal. Surgeons performed an operation called thoracoplasty, in which consecutive ribs were removed to allow the chest wall to collapse inward. The operation was incredibly disfiguring, leaving the patient with a sunken, deformed chest. Even more frightening was that these extensive operations, sometimes involving nine rib resections, were done under injections of a local anesthetic (such as novocaine), since intratracheal anesthesia wasn't invented until 1930. Another type of collapse therapy that was utilized was plombage, in which an inert material was inserted into the chest cavity to fill the empty space. In the 1940s, plastic Ping-Pong balls were the material of choice, and the procedure was known as Ping-Pong ball plombage. Say that three times fast.

The truth be told, if it wasn't for the development of general anesthesia delivered through an endotracheal tube, the field of cardiothoracic surgery wouldn't exist today. The first open lung cases, such as lung resections for cancer or infection, had to be done in a negative pressure chamber to keep the lung from collapsing and straining the heart. This was a hermetically sealed box that enclosed not only the patient but the entire OR team as well, leaving just the patient's head outside so that he/she could breathe. On October 16, 1846, Dr. Morton (a dentist) and Dr. Warren (a surgeon) put a patient "to sleep" using ether as a general anesthetic and performed a twenty-five-minute operation. This was done at the Massachusetts General Hospital in an operating theater since known as the Ether Dome, and the day is still celebrated at the MGH as Ether Day.

Despite the advent of anesthesia, lung operations were still very crude compared to what I do today. To resect the lung, either a small portion or its entirety, the lung was ligated and then left to slough out of the chest opening over the course of two weeks. Presently, lung resections can be done using a minimally invasive approach known as video-assisted thoracoscopic surgery. Several small one-inch "keyhole" incisions are used and the operation is done with a camera and scope. Usually the patients can go home the next day. Dr. Vista and I used to marvel at the way "they used to do it" and wonder what the future of lung surgery would hold.

Dr. Vista's favorite subject to discuss, though, was the history of heart surgery, and we would spend much time talking about the cardiac cowboys who roamed the cardiac frontier looking for adventure. He said, "You had to be fearless, willing to do anything and operate on anybody, and be a little bit crazy to be a heart surgeon back then. Brass balls, that's what it took. The patients you got to operate on were at death's door and, frankly, you really didn't know which side of the door they were on. When it came to needing heart surgery, even the smallest of procedures, it was usually a last-ditch effort and all other treatment modalities had failed. Poor bastards."

The heart was (and still is) felt to be the seat of the soul. In the late 1800s and early 1900s, surgeons didn't operate on the heart because they feared that if the chest was opened and the heart exposed, the soul would escape from the body, resulting in the patient's death. Pioneering surgeons who so much as thought about operating on the heart were considered, according to one legendary quote, "foolhardy," and in doing so "a surgeon should lose the respect of his peers."

Heart surgeons evolved from thoracic surgeons, and surgery of the heart began as a necessity to treat chest injuries that occurred during times of war. The surgeon Ludwig Rehn is credited with the first successful heart operation when in 1896 he repaired a stab wound in the right ventricle of a soldier. Some of the greatest and most lasting achievements in heart surgery, however, were the development of coronary artery bypass surgery and the achievement of successful heart transplantation.

To even begin to conceptualize bypass surgery, the coronary arteries needed to be visualized. Dr. Vista used to love to tell the story of "that crazy bastard" Dr. Werner Forssmann, who in 1929 performed a cardiac catheterization—on himself! After tying his medical assistant to an OR table so she couldn't stop him, this German urologist, using a mirror, actually cut open his own left arm at the crease of his elbow, located the brachial vein, and then inserted a thin filamentous urologic catheter, a ureteral catheter. He threaded the catheter up his arm and into the right-sided heart chambers. As Dr. Vista tells it, Forssmann then walked upstairs to the radiology department, with the catheter protruding from his arm, to take an X-ray and confirm his successful catheter placement. Such is the spirit and drive of medical pioneers!

The bread and butter of what we do as cardiac surgeons is coronary artery bypass grafting, or CABG for short. We sew blood vessels to blood vessels to bring a new blood supply to the heart where there is a shortage owing to an arterial blockage. We call it laying pipe and will greet each other at the OR board where the cases are posted by asking, "Whatareyadoin' today?" Answer: "Just laying pipe, my friend, just laying pipe."

But the first CABG procedures weren't anything like what we do today. The Beck procedure, named after Dr. Claude S. Beck (1894–1971), who, incidentally, was a surgeon at my alma mater, (Case) Western Reserve University, involved abrading the heart with talcum powder and asbestos. These abrasions would then heal themselves by growing new vessels into the area, a revascularization process known as developing collateral circulation. Dr. Arthur M. Vineberg (1903–1988) next developed a procedure in 1946 whereby the left internal mammary artery, which courses down the inside of the front of your chest wall, was sewn into a tunnel in the muscle of the heart. The branches of the artery were left to bleed freely into the muscle, and this blood seeped between the muscle fibers to bring in a new blood supply to the area. Following this procedure, for the next twenty years or so, blockage in the coronary arteries was treated by opening these tiny arteries and scooping out the calcium and fat buildup that caused the blockage. The technique, still used in peripheral vascular surgery such as carotid artery surgery, is known as endarterectomy. It wasn't until the early 1960s, when Dr. Vista was in training, that surgeons started sewing peripheral arteries and veins directly to the heart's native coronary arteries.

But by far, Dr. Vista's fondest story was about the early days of heart transplantation when his overly ambitious friend, "Chris" Barnard, performed the first successful heart transplant in Cape Town, South Africa. He liked to call Christiaan Barnard "Chris" as a way to remind you that he knew him personally. On December 3, 1967, Dr. Barnard took the heart from a twenty-five-year-old woman, Denise Darvall, who was brain dead from a car accident, and implanted it into Louis Washansky, a forty-five-year-old man bedridden with heart failure. He lived for eighteen days. The publicity of this event was far-reaching, and overnight Christiaan Barnard became a household name and a celebrity.

One month later, he performed another heart transplant on a dentist, who lived for two years. After an initial flurry of heart transplants over the next four years, heart transplants all but ceased in 1971 because of universally poor outcomes owing to rejection. One surgeon didn't despair, though. Dr. Norman Shumway at Stanford University Hospital kept the transplant torch burning by continuing to improve the technique of heart transplantation through his endless experimental work and research. I had the honor of meeting him once when I was at Stanford to interview for a transplant fellowship position. He was truly one of the legendary greats of cardiac surgery, but to meet him you wouldn't know it. He was such a sweet and unassuming man. He showed up at my interview wearing green plaid golf knickers, a white polo shirt, and a matching golf beret complete with pom-pom. I thought for a minute that I was being interviewed by Payne Stewart. His eyes were youthful and inquisitive. His manner was very gentle. As I sat in his office, I couldn't help but be amazed. Because of this one man's unfailing efforts and the invention of the powerful anti-rejection medication cyclosporine, in 1976, heart transplantation has become a routinely performed procedure.

When we finished reminiscing about cardiac surgery, Dr. Vista would ask, "You wanna walk around?" This was his way of asking me to see his patients with him. He would never ask me to "make rounds," since this was strictly forbidden. So we would take a walk around the hospital and just "happen" to wind up in a postoperative patient's room. Rounds with him were a trip, let me tell you. When we hit the patient floor, you could see the look of dread from the nurses, whom he referred to as "white-coat-wearing, clipboard-carrying castrating bitches." When he approached, they would collectively scatter in front of him the way pigeons scatter when chased by a terrorizing two-year-old.

He did things the old-fashioned way, the good ol' boys' way. For example, he would enter a patient's room, tap her deftly up and down her back, a technique known as "percussing," and decide, without the use of a stethoscope or chest X-ray, that she had pleural effusion (fluid around the lung) that needed to be drained off. He would then take a large needle, which he just happened to have in his pocket, pick a spot on her back, and shove the needle in. My job was to get plastic tubing and a glass bottle, which contained a vacuum seal to drain the collected fluid into, in the space of time it took him to sink his needle. This sent me running around the room like a chicken with its head cut off. When the fluid was done draining, he withdrew the needle and, I kid you not, opened his brown leather billfold, took out a Band-Aid (which I assume he regularly carried), and slapped it on the site of the puncture to serve as a "dressing." Nowadays, there is a whole "process" for draining a pleural effusion that includes an X-ray, an ultrasound, possibly even a computerized axial tomography (CAT) scan, as well as discussion with the patient outlining the procedure and its risks and benefits. This is followed by a consent form complete with an unbiased witness signature. Then there is the prepping, the draping, the local anesthesia, the setting up of an entire lung-tapping kit. The procedure culminates with an elaborate and well-placed surgical dressing, which, despite your best efforts, usually falls off as soon as the patient sits up. More often than not, the whole thing is done in a radiology suite by a radiologist or pulmonary medicine specialist. And we wonder why health care costs are on the rise?

When I think back to the first day that I met Dr. Vista, I am amazed that he ever let me into his inner circle in the first place. It was July of 1990, and like any young surgeon in training, I was greener than green and saw my job as just trying to stay out of everyone's way and not kill anyone. But trouble always seems to find me.

· · ·

Sometimes I wish I had never responded to the yelling for help that came from the recovery room that day. And what if

I hadn't? Dr. Vista probably never would have noticed me despite the fact that I would spend the next six years of my life at his hospital. Forgetting that I was supposed to stay out of the way, I headed into the recovery room. There was a patient in full cardiac arrest following a complete removal of his left lung (known as a pneumonectomy). CPR was in progress, but the recovery room team was having no luck in getting the patient back. Instead of jumping into the fray (a wise decision at the time), I stepped back from the scene and took a good look at what was happening. I saw that the patient's chest tube was exiting from the side of his left chest, as it should, but I couldn't see the bottle into which it was draining. The bottle had been pushed behind the ventilator, which was next to the patient's bed. So I followed the chest drain to its origin, as you would if you were following an extension cord back to the electrical socket to see if it's plugged in. When I finally got to the drainage bottle hidden behind the ventilator, I saw, to my horror, that the bottle was full of blood and, in fact, had fallen over. Blood was pooling on the floor beneath the bed—thick, dark red blood—and a lot of it. I knew, even as an intern, that the only way to save this patient was to get control of whatever had cut loose in his chest. For the next few maneuvers that I did, I need to plead temporary insanity—I truly had no idea what I was doing. It was like having an out-of-body experience. My arms and legs were in motion, my mouth was saying things, but I was completely removed from the events. I was scared out of my wits. I just started dragging the bed, patient and all, back to the nearest unoccupied operating room. Luckily, I dragged the bed to the OR where the case had been performed. The operating room hadn't been "turned over," meaning that all the surgical instruments were

still out and available. With the patient still lying in his
recovery room bed, I saw my right hand take a No. 10 blade
scalpel and slice along the patient's freshly sutured chest incision. I saw myself attempt to place a chest retractor into the
wound to spread the chest incision wide open. Because my
hands were shaking violently, I next saw myself drop the retractor onto the OR floor. My hands then picked up the retractor from the floor and, without wiping it off, replaced it
into the wound. (Remember, the patient is dying here.) I saw
my left hand grab a suction catheter and suck out the remaining blood from the chest. I then saw both hands put a
large clamp across the pulmonary artery from whence the
blood was pouring.

The pulmonary artery, you should know, is a big bad artery. It's a very friable structure, which is to say, it is flimsy and
tears easily. The pulmonary artery carries all the blood from
the right side of the heart to the lungs to get oxygen. You can
bleed to death from the open end of it in a matter of a few
heartbeats. We now have vascular stapling devices that ele-
gantly staple off the pulmonary artery with little effort on the
surgeon's part. When I was an intern, however, the pulmonary
artery, when transected for complete lung removal, was closed
with one or two large metal clips and/or oversewn with suture.
If the clips came off or a suture broke when a patient coughed
violently while on the ventilator after surgery, then you would
wind up with a chest tube bottle full of blood and a patient in
full cardiac arrest.

Once I got control of the bleeding, the anesthesiologist
could "catch up" by pouring blood quickly into the patient to
replace what had drained out. Dr. Vista arrived in the OR (did
I mention that this was his patient?) cursing and screaming.

All I could make out was "What the fuck is that nurse doing touching my patient?" "That nurse," the anesthesiologist said, "is a doctor and she just saved your patient's life." Dr. Vista grunted and said in his usually curt manner, "Finish it." Although he meant for me to close up the patient, I could have sworn he said, "You're finished," as in "Pack your bags, dearie, because you're going home to mamma and you ain't gonna be a surgeon no more."

At this point you're probably wondering why I call this man my mentor. Well, for starters, he was the first surgeon not to look at me as if I had a third eye in the middle of my forehead when I said that I wanted to be a heart surgeon. He encouraged me to go into the field that few women had entered. This unwavering encouragement kept my passion for heart surgery alive even as the work itself became increasingly exhausting and overwhelming. Second, he was a slick surgeon. He could "shuck a vein" (his words) in five minutes flat using nothing other than a scalpel. This vein-harvesting procedure entailed stripping out the vein of a leg from ankle to thigh (depending how much length is needed) so it could be used as a conduit for a bypass graft. An extensive incision is made in the skin all the way up the leg and then you dissect down to the saphenous vein and meticulously identify, tie off, and cut each of the many dozen branches that may be present so that you are left with a long tube of vein. The procedure, done in this manner, can take thirty to forty-five minutes. (Nowadays, through a procedure known as endoscopic vein harvest, we can take this length of vein out using a single one-inch incision. Well, at least my physician's assistant, Matt, can. He's a whiz.) Back then, I would marvel at how Dr. Vista could do it with such speed and alacrity. He used quick short strokes with his knife and looked like a sushi chef trimming a delicate piece of toro. He was equally fast with every other part of the cardiac operation and I, for one, personally admired his combination of speed and accuracy.

· · ·

I haven't spoken to Dr. Vista in a few years and so I recently called him. He's since retired to a beautiful gated community to enjoy life with his family. I asked him if he still calls people rat-fuckers. "I haven't much occasion to these days," he replied with a laugh. It seems as though he has mellowed with time.

After catching up on what we have each been doing, we lapsed into our same old habit of reminiscing about the good old days of cardiothoracic surgery. A time of intrigue and discovery. A time of fearlessness and bravery. Secretly, he and I hope that we each leave a small footprint on the cardiac frontier.

I would really like to see him, but he isn't too inclined to come out here to "La La Land," which is what he calls the entire state of California. The last thing he said to me on the phone was "You are my greatest accomplishment, a story unto itself."

7

Fire and Ice

"I'M ON FIRE!" I THOUGHT IT AT THE SAME TIME I SAID IT. The nurse standing to my left in the OR remained completely oblivious to this fact, her mask neatly tied around her dainty nose and mouth in a speak-no-evil kind of way. The OR, cold and brilliantly lit, was in complete disarray. Laparotomy pads and gauze sponges were strewn all over the floor. A mound of unused, contaminated drapes loomed in the far corner. The clear plastic tubing used for cardiopulmonary bypass was a tangled mess of knotted hoses draped over the OR table. The surgical instruments, usually lined up in a neat, orderly row, were haphazardly covering the Mayo stand in a careless manner. And the yelling, the din of everyone in the OR—the surgeons, nurses, anesthesiologists, technicians, assistants—speaking at once was deafening.

I don't know which was worse: the disheveled OR, the hell breaking loose around me, or the simple fact that my hand was on fire. I kept watching my hand to see if I could indeed see the flames as they consumed my size 7 surgical glove, but since pure alcohol burns clean, I could only feel the glove searing into my skin as it melted upon my hand.

"For Christ's sake, someone put me out!" I yelled to no one specifically. To everyone in general.

To my horror, I saw the flames lick the patient's skin as well as the surgical drapes. It was spreading. The fire was spreading. Imperceptible at first but then, most decisively. It was on a mission: to burn everything in its path. Me→the drapes→the patient→the anesthesiologist→the OR staff→the floor→the walls→the lights→the ceiling→the door→the OR hallway→past the front desk→to the patient corridors→into the hospital itself. The hospital in its entirety.

The No. 10 blade scalpel glowed red-white hot as it lay next to the incision I had made in the patient's groin. The patient, a woman in her sixties with known heart disease, was in full cardiac arrest and we had to get on the heart-lung machine NOW! While my surgical partner was opening the chest, I had been dissecting out the femoral artery and vein so we could quickly attach her to the heart-lung machine through these large vessels. Then the fire started. The nurses had hastily prepped the arresting patient with a solution that contained 74 percent isopropyl alcohol and draped the patient without allowing three minutes for the alcohol to evaporate. When I used the Bovie, an electrocautery device, it sparked and ignited the alcohol. When the fire got out of control, I knew I had to do something. I knew that I had to stop it before it came in contact with the oxygen being administered to the patient and killed us all. But how? I had no bucket of water. No blankets. I looked around the room for something to help me douse the flames. Nothing. There was nothing. And no one, other than me, realized what was actually happening. No one saw the clear flames shimmer across the blue drapes. No one felt the burning pain. They were all completely absorbed in the full cardiac arrest.

I then did something that, in retrospect, was either incredibly heroic or incredibly stupid. I thrust my entire upper body upon the flames, depriving them of oxygen, and put the fire out. No oxygen. No flames.

When I say that I put the fire out, what I really mean is that I put the patient out, not myself. I was still on fire; my hand and now the cuff of my surgical gown were ablaze. I knew that if I waved my hand wildly I would only incite the flames and so I calmly and slowly put my hand and wrist under my armpit and smothered them.

Within minutes, the entire hospital had heard about the fire. Within an hour, an RCA, or root cause analysis, meeting was called. When something untoward occurs in a hospital, it is identified as a sentinel event. The Sentinel Event Committee, formed by a chosen group of doctors, administrators, and risk-management personnel as well as the staff involved in the actual event, reviews the event and tries to find the causal factors in an effort to prevent it from happening again. Often, this RCA meeting is quite helpful. A protective mechanism, it's the hospital's way of licking its wounds and healing itself by changing processes to improve performance and reduce risk. It is also a CYA move because the Sentinel Event Committee minutes are written during an RCA meeting and cannot be subpoenaed by lawyers and are therefore undiscoverable if a patient sues. Sometimes, however, it is more like a lynch mob.

Not that anyone at the RCA meeting cared, but because

I had reacted so quickly, neither the patient nor I sustained any significant burns, although I carry a small scar at the base of my left thumb. At the RCA meeting, we reviewed what happened and, as a result, changed the way we prep patients for an emergency procedure. It was interesting that not one committee member remarked about the fact that I had put the patient out *first* and myself *second*. To accomplish this you have to override every self-preservation instinct that tells you to take care of yourself first and the guy next to you second. But the patient comes first. Patients always come first. It is our oath and our honor as doctors. It is part of our instinctual behavior. We are healers and rescuers.

As we filed out of the room at the meeting's conclusion, the anesthesiologist who had been in the OR during the fire came up behind me and whispered, "I've never seen anyone on fire be so calm."

"Oh, have you seen a lot of people catch on fire?" I winked at him and smiled. "Happens to me a lot."

I have learned over the years that staying calm in the operating room is an important tool—just as important as our suture and our scalpel. A surgeon is not necessarily born with this tool. She must learn it. She must earn it.

The surgeon whom I learned it and earned it from was a real prick. But my God, could this man operate. When he wasn't doing open heart surgery, he was playing piano, and his limber hands would glide along the surgical field like a concert pianist. He was quick and precise. I admired him, envied him, and hated him all at the same time. If I saw him today on a street corner, I don't know if I would shake his hand or punch him in the stomach.

I never saw him lose his cool in the OR. I would watch

patients bleed out beneath his hands and he didn't show the slightest tremor. His voice never cracked. He would just calmly fix the problem like he was darning a sock. He used to yell at me in the OR all the time. He'd do it precisely at the moment when I was taking some crucial, incredibly difficult stitch. Like someone screaming an obscenity from the PGA gallery when Tiger Woods was beginning his downswing, he did this to unnerve me. To see if I would flinch. To test my focus. To upset my balance. Sometimes he would even rap my knuckles with the backside of a DeBakey forceps when yelling alone didn't work. I don't know if it was because he saw potential in me or he just got some sadistic enjoyment out of torturing me. I do know, however, that he made me learn to be a better surgeon. A calm, focused, unflinchable surgeon. I learned it *and* I earned it.

Under his tutelage, I became ice in the OR. Cold. Hard. Ice. You could see through me to my core, but you couldn't get to me. You couldn't hold me in your hands very long or I would freeze your marrow. Ice. A thick block. The kind that doesn't melt in the heat of a Maine summer. The kind that doesn't crack beneath a skater's blade. The kind that doesn't shatter when struck by an ice pick. Ice. Cold. Hard. Ice.

They actually nicknamed me that in my residency. Not "Ice Queen," since that would have a different connotation altogether. Just "Ice." I think, perhaps, that I became this icy thing because the expectation of my colleagues was that as a female, I would be more like Jell-O in the OR. Soft, quivering, unsteady. I needed to get as far away from this female stereotype as possible. Maybe my torturer knew this as well. Maybe that's why he made me ice.

So now, when the going gets tough in the OR, I get cold.

Ice cold. But not in a mean-spirited way. I just get very quiet and very focused. I go somewhere deep inside myself to a place that is mine alone. A place that is quiet, calm, and cold. I begin speaking in a manner that is very soft, very courteous, and very slow.

"Would you please hand me a 4-0 Prolene, single-armed with a pledget?"

"Thank you. And next I'll take a free pledget on a short hemostat."

"That's great. Can you please have two more available for me? Thanks."

"Terrific. And now I'll need the next one backhanded, please."

And so the pleases and thank-yous go, one after another, attached to some crucial command that is not spoken harshly or with a raised voice but rather in a soft, cool monotone. By now the nurses know that when I start saying "please" and "thank you," the proverbial shit must be hitting the fan.

Each surgeon is unique in the way in which he or she handles pressure in the OR. One surgeon I knew would hum Mozart loudly when things went utterly wrong. I've seen others scream, yell, and throw instruments, which completely unglues everyone in the OR and only serves to jeopardize the life of the patient. I once had to calm a surgeon down in the operating room by head-butting him across the OR table because he had gone completely off the deep end.

Ice serves a purpose for me. It provides a place in my soul from which I can maintain my composure during a crisis. The nice thing about my ice is that in a process of sublimation, I can completely change from this cold solid to my warm, airy, effusive self when the crisis has been averted and I come out from beneath the OR lights.

It's just me again.

The surgeon who hugs her patients.

The surgeon who loves her patients.

A surgeon with warmth,

Fire,

And Ice.

8

Sex and the Surgeon

I WOULD LIKE TO TAKE THIS OPPORTUNITY TO DISPEL SOME of the misconceptions surrounding sex and the surgeon. We are not, for example, sex-starved fiends who duck into the nearest janitorial closet or medical supply room to have yearning sex with a nurse half our age among the mop buckets and bedpans. We do not fall head over heels in love with our patients and fantasize about putting in their urinary catheters while they are under an anesthetic. Nor do we engage in after-hours hookups with our patients' family members in our offices so that we can split the life insurance policy when they succumb to their disease.

Television has always set the bar high for surgeons' sexual prowess and I for one would like to set the record straight so as not to disappoint my next conquest. (Oh. That's right. I'm married.) Someone once described *Grey's Anatomy* as "*ER* meets *Sex and the City*." I'd say that is a pretty fair assessment. My mom religiously watches *Grey's Anatomy* and every other medical television drama and now firmly believes:

> A. *You can drop an organ on the floor. Pick it up. Wash it off. And transplant it into the patient as if nothing happened.*
>
> B. *I must be a slut.*

Thanks, ABC.

Now, I'm not saying that I am an angel. Nor am I saying that things like this don't go on in a hospital. I'm not and they do. Just as they probably do at every other workplace. As surgeons, we spend the majority of the day in the hospital, and yes, it becomes our home away from home. In fact, we have a commonly used expression for being in the hospital— we call it being in-house. As in, "Hey, are you in-house tonight?" Which translates to "Hey, are you in the hospital on call all night tonight?" When asked if you are in the hospital, your answer wouldn't be "Yeah, I'm here;" it would be "Yeah, I'm in-house." And so it goes without saying that if you are spending more time in "the house" locked in among the sick and the sicker, rather than "your house," which is where your TV is located, you may have to hook up here or go without.

But sex for the surgeon, especially when you are a resident or fellow essentially living in the hospital, is a release. It momentarily takes you away from the suffering and the sickness. You feel alive among the dead. You feel the pleasure among the pain. But I still don't know why television portrays us as a bunch of superficial bed hoppers. Perhaps that's entertainment.

One of the other myths to dispel is the relationship between attending doctors and the medical students, interns, and residents with whom they interact. The relationship is that of a teacher-student relationship, and as such, the students are forbidden fruit. You cannot, therefore, cherry-pick among the interns and residents for your next illicit affair. Hospitals have codes of conduct regarding this. Again, I'm not saying it doesn't happen; I'm saying that it is regarded as taboo, like kissing your brother or sister. Despite this, on television we, the surgeons, are at the forefront of seducing our pupils.

I usually keep my head down and move about my day, and interludes often go unnoticed by me. I have, on occasion, caught a colleague or two with "someone" who wasn't a spouse. I have also seen nurses being openly flirtatious with doctors and vice versa. But honestly, it doesn't come close to what the public believes goes on in hospitals, a veritable den of iniquity. Sorry to disappoint.

As a woman in the world of medicine, it is particularly difficult to remain above reproach on this issue of sex and the surgeon. I think people just assume that I am sleeping with every male nurse or colleague I speak to. To this end, I will always leave my office door open when meeting with anyone with an X and a Y chromosome. I have a nurse in the room with me when examining a male patient. And any blatant flirtation by a colleague is met with a pathetically uninterested blank stare. This is because, yes, I have been hit on by male patients, nurses, residents, and colleagues, and yes, it is taboo.

While we're on the subject of *sex,* I think it prudent to discuss *sexism.* I am going to try to do this, however, without sounding like I have a permanent chip on my acromion (in nonmedical-speak, shoulder). For the record, sexism is alive and well in the field of medicine. Ask any female doctor. It's our dirty little secret. Now, as long as you stay within the branches of medicine that are traditionally female—pediatrics, OB-GYN, plastic surgery, dermatology—you're probably all right. But try cutting a swath into the nontraditional fields and you had better watch it, girlfriend.

I've tried to stay above the fray on this, but it's awfully hard to when you finally get your first job and you are paid less than half the salary of your male surgical colleagues, you are forced to sit in the secretarial pool in a cubicle instead of an office, and as recently as last week you were told by a male cardiologist that he simply cannot refer patients to you because he "just can't get past the fact that you're a woman." And one wonders why the glass ceiling of medicine has been bloodied mostly by the women who have hit it.

Sure, I've tried to just fit in. That's always been my strategy. Not to stand out. Not to differentiate myself because I am a woman. I shared a call room with the guys I was in fellowship with, didn't I? But there's something unequal going on when the male OR locker room door says SURGEONS and the female OR locker room door says NURSES. I don't know. Maybe I'm just being overly sensitive.

There were three distinct moments in my career when I almost quit, and all three moments had to do with sexism and sexual harassment. Death, fatigue, sickness—none of these drove me to the edge. But when I was put down as a woman, I felt my knees buckle at the precipice and nearly went over the side. It truly rocked my world.

The first event occurred when I was a fledgling surgeon in training. I was in the OR with an attending who had a reputation for being quite the ladies' man. I had always made it a point to steer clear of him. Perfect body, perfect hair, and the fact that he always leaned into a woman when he spoke to her were the telltale signs that said to me, in blinking neon lights, "Keep away." I found myself assigned to do a simple case with him—a bronchoscopy with brush biopsy. The patient was suspected of having a cancer in the lumen of one of his bronchi, which are the tubes that carry air to and from the lungs. We were going to insert a lighted scope into the bronchi and then brush the sides of the airway with a tiny toothbrush-like apparatus that we insert, under direct vision, through the scope. This enables us to sample or biopsy the wall to look for a lurking cancer. To get an adequate sample, you have to move the brush quickly in and out of the scope much like you would move a pipe cleaner in and out of a pipe to scrape its walls.

I began the procedure by standing at the head of the OR table so I could introduce the scope into the patient's trachea and guide it distally. Initially, the attending guided me through the procedure with verbal instruction, but soon he said, "Here, let me help you" and moved in behind me so that both his arms were around me holding the scope alongside mine and his chin was on my left shoulder. This procedure is really a single-person operation, and the more he pressed his body against me, the more I inched closer to the patient until I was pinned between the edge of the OR table and the lecher. I tried to stay calm. I tried to just focus on the procedure at hand. It was when I began to do the brush biopsy that he whispered, none too softly, in my left ear, "No, no. You're not doing it right. Move the brush in and out faster. Shorter strokes. Like you would if you were jerking me off." I felt his weight crush me. My body and my spirit. My abdomen tensed with pain and disgust. I looked up from the scope just long enough to see the scrub nurse leer at me, her eyes speaking to me in a sarcastic tone: "Are you and your *boyfriend* done having sex in my OR?" I was so young. So innocent. So hurt. The tension in my abdomen took over my body until I was a rigid board frozen there in his embrace. Every fiber of my being told me to elbow him in the gut as hard as I could and get the hell out. Run away. Quit. Hide. I felt ashamed. Dirty, used, and ashamed. It was my fault somehow, wasn't it? Did I lead him on? Was I in any way suggestive in the OR? He didn't respect me as a woman and he certainly didn't respect me as a surgeon. To him, I wasn't a budding physician wanting to immerse myself in learning. To him, I was a toy. A Barbie doll wearing a surgical mask.

And what do I do now? Tell on him? Rat him out for his vulgarity? Right. And lose my job. In the early '90s, as a woman, you just shut up and took it like a man. I have never told that story to anyone, and now, essentially, I've told *every-one*. And yet I feel no relief. The pain is as real today as the day it happened. It still sickens me. It makes me bow my head in shame.

The second incident occurred later on in my training, and although I was a little older and wiser, the sting of it still pierced my armor and I almost quit. It happened at the con-clusion of a particularly difficult and rewarding surgical case that I had done with a young attending. To this day, I can't recall what the case involved exactly since the memory of it is obscured by what was said to me in the OR that day. The attending surgeon was giddy with the excitement of having just done a terrific job saving a patient's life. I, too, was beaming with pride at having helped him and played what I believed to be an important part. At the height of my pride, that's when he did it. That's when he snatched away my pride as if it were a trophy I hadn't earned by leaning over and saying, "Do you have any idea how much I want to fuck you right now?"

When I was a kid, I had a favorite apple tree in the orchard that I liked to climb. It was a young, tall tree that produced the best Red Delicious apples. Unlike the wizened old Golden Delicious trees that were a cinch to climb, my tree took quite the skill. Once, and only once, I took a terrible fall from high up in my tree. I hit the ground solidly upon my back and knocked the wind out of myself. I remember feeling the pain of the fall followed by the urge to exhale, exhale, exhale, exhale. I couldn't catch my breath. I couldn't inhale. Just exhaling and exhaling and exhaling until there was no breath left in my body. I thought I was going to die right there on the ground, covered in rotten Red Delicious apples with two of my brothers standing over me.

That's *exactly* how it felt when he said those words to me. When he took my pride, self-esteem, and breath away with one sexist comment. I couldn't breathe. I was suffocating right there in front of him. There was no air. Everything was leaving my body. My passion, my joy, my desire to continue my training as a surgeon—it was all being ripped from my being like having the wind knocked out of me. I put my head down. I closed my eyes and thought, "Inhale, inhale, inhale."

I wanted to say something. I didn't. I couldn't. I wanted to say, "Look at me. Look at me, you horrible man. See me. But don't look any deeper than my plastic factory-molded exterior, because if you do, you might just find a surgeon waiting to emerge and stand confidently across from you at the OR table. No, don't look any deeper because that would ruin your fantasy. Your Barbie doll in a surgical mask fantasy." Again, fearing for my job, I kept my mouth shut and just took it.

The third time I nearly quit tested the limits of the level of sexism that I could withstand and not throw it all away. I had so much to lose this time because I was almost finished with my training. The light at the end of the tunnel was fast approaching.

I finished a case with an attending surgeon who was a division chief. Since I had done a particularly good job, he asked me if I wanted to go out to the surgery waiting room with him and talk to the patient's family. My God, I was so delighted. Usually only the attending spoke to the family after surgery and I was so pleased that he would recognize me in this way. I felt like part of the team. I felt like I belonged. Like I was one of the surgeons. Like I fit in. Not different because I was a woman but the same because I was a surgeon on equal footing.

We greeted the patient's wife and his two daughters, who were nearly my age. I stood by the attending's side like a second in command while he told them how well the procedure went. He didn't acknowledge me until his report to the family was nearing the end. "And Kathy, here, she did a hell of a job," he said, and then slapped me hard on my ass like a football player hitting a teammate after a touchdown. The strike was so hard, in fact, that I lurched forward toward the family and everyone in the waiting room heard it. The three women in front of me had this look of shock. I could see that they were searching my face quickly to read my reaction. The sting of my bottom was not as great as the sting of the tears just beginning to form in my eyes or the sting of my lower lip as I crushed it between my teeth. Despite this, however, I held my composure like a weight lifter during a clean-and-jerk lift. I steadied myself and did not allow them to read my reaction. I just stood there like a wooden soldier. Just when I felt my body start to give way beneath the weight of disgust and shame that was bearing down upon me, I feigned a gesture that my pager had gone off and headed out of the waiting room to pretend to answer it.

I went straight to the nearest women's bathroom and kicked in every door of every stall. I wanted to tear the place apart while letting all of my pent-up anger spew from my body. Why did I have to take this, the ultimate ridicule, the ultimate kick in the teeth? Because I had no recourse, that's why. Although I wanted to quit, I just couldn't throw it all away. I wanted to be a heart surgeon so badly, more than anything else in my life. Like any patient facing surgery, I weighed the risks and benefits of my situation. I felt the benefits of keeping quiet outweighed the risks of telling and the risks of quitting. I weighed the pain and humiliation I felt at that moment in time against all that I had accomplished to date.

In the end, like all the other times, I let it go. A red balloon on a string; I just let it go. Let the incident soar away from me until I could no longer see it in the stratosphere. I did nothing and said nothing and let my career move along its inevitable path. So is there a grudge here to hold? Probably, but not by me. I consider myself a path paver for other woman who choose to go into cardiac surgery. Sure, the path I paved has a few potholes—what rugged path doesn't? Being a pioneer has a price and I paid that price so that others might follow my lead. My only hope is that somehow I have made it easier for the next woman and have opened a few doors that would otherwise remain closed.

To this end, I have begun mentoring young girls who

may be considering a career in medicine, because I do believe that it is still a noble profession. The fact that I get to go to work each day and help complete strangers is the most rewarding of careers. How many people do that day in and day out? Just help people. And yet, I am taken aback sometimes when I am in a classroom of young children my son's age and ask, "Can girls be doctors?" and hear some noes among the answers. Children just don't see women in those roles and I wish that were different, because I think children grow up with a prejudice toward women in traditionally male roles.

Because of this, I am trying to raise two boys to believe that women not only can be mommies but can also be more than mommies if they choose—that woman can be firefighters, police officers, pilots, and captains of industry. They can even be heart surgeons if they so desire. I was vindicated the other day when my son Nicholas was practicing writing his full name. He wanted to write mine and I told him it was Kathy Elizabeth Magliato, MD. After carefully writing the letters, he asked what MD meant. Before I could answer he said, "Oh, I know what it means—Mommy Doctor."

"Yes," I said, "that's exactly what it means."

9

One of the Girls

T HE HARDEST THING TO DO IS TO BE ONE OF THE GIRLS
when you're one of the guys. When I was a kid, I was a total
tomboy. I hung around with my three younger brothers and
played with G.I. Joes and trucks instead of Barbies and Easy-
Bake ovens with my older sister. My favorite thing to do as a
kid was to climb trees, and I once tackled a weeping willow
that would give most kids a head injury or, at the very least,
an arm broken in two places.

I even looked like a boy—skinny, no boobs, short hair,
and dressed in carpenter pants and construction boots. I never
wore dresses and my mom used to tease me and say that when
I got married I would wear jeans under my wedding dress. I
could beat up any kid on the block and defended my younger
brothers against any bully with the tenacity of a pit bull. I was
one tough chick.

My enduring friendship with my brothers made it possible
for me to feel very much at home in such a male-dominated

profession as cardiac surgery. I am truly grateful to my brothers for teaching me how to work and play well with the men and boys in my life. And especially for teaching me how to hold my own.

The American Board of Thoracic Surgery was established in October of 1948. It is the certifying body that administers the exams for cardiothoracic surgeons to become board certified following their training. It is necessary for a heart surgeon to become board certified in order to practice in a hospital. Since 1948 the board has awarded approximately 7,400 certificates (my certificate is No. 6276). In 1961 the board certified its first woman, Dr. Nina Starr Braunwald. From 1961 to 2008, of those 7,400 certificates, only 180 have been awarded to women. With so few female cardiothoracic surgeons, I have worked exclusively with male colleagues.

. . .

Although it has always been a struggle for me to maintain my femininity and my nurturing side while trying to be a tough heart surgeon, this struggle is essential to who I am as a person and as a doctor. I need to be ice in the OR and still be able to sit on the edge of patients' beds and hold their hands to comfort them when I tell them that their metastatic lung cancer is not resectable. Great doctors have both toughness and compassion. But being soft on the outside and hard on the inside takes a delicate balance. It seems as though I can maintain this balance quite well with patients, but with personal relationships . . . it's a whole other story.

For the most part, I maintain a "one of the boys" attitude, both in how I act and how I dress, when I am around my male colleagues. I am chummy but never flirtatious. No subject is off-limits in the OR during a case no matter how crass or locker room–ish it might be. The only thing I can't do is hold my own during a conversation about sports. In general, men are at ease with me. If, however, I wear an above-the-knee skirt to work because I have managed to find the time to shave my legs, my IQ precipitously drops 60 points in the eyes of my male colleagues. They start acting weird, almost coy, when I come to work dressed like a girl and they treat me like I'm dumb. So I don't. I dress conservatively—mostly pants and long skirts. Makeup is a must but not overly done. No jewelry. Ironically, though, the other day I saw a male surgeon wearing one-carat diamond studs in both ears and I thought, "Maybe I should polish my jewels and live a little." My next thought, however, was "Nah. I'd probably lose a silver hoop earring in someone's chest and that would be an awful mess."

My relationship with female colleagues, specifically nurses, however, has been more difficult. It always backfires on me when I try to be "one of the girls," and yet I long to have successful relationships with women at the hospital. I can't quite figure out why it never works. After all, I have amazing relationships with other women in my life. My sister, for example, is my best friend in spite of the fact that we never got along as kids. I have girlfriends outside of work who are more than just shopping buddies. But trying to have a friendship with a nurse—no way. If I am too friendly with them and try to be one of the girls, then they don't take me seriously as a doctor. They let my orders slide. If I get upset with them about a patient's care, they are instantly hurt, as if I have betrayed them somehow. There is such a double standard: My male colleagues can outright scream at a female nurse and they are thought of as "assertive" or as "just keeping the patient's best interest in mind." If I were to yell at a nurse, I'd be labeled as a *bitch* and would lose my job. I was recently criticized by a nurse for not "standing up for her" when a male colleague was harsh with her regarding the management of a patient. She said, "We're women, we need to stick together." But playing the gender card has never worked for me. So I stay in my comfort zone of being one of the boys at work and forfeit a friendship with a nurse.

My relationships with men exclusive of those with whom I work have been the most difficult for me to maintain. The fastest way for me to get rid of a guy in a bar is to tell him what I do for a living. He either becomes instantly intimidated or horribly grossed out. Perhaps he's wondering if I have blood under my fingernails or thinking that "I'm a heart surgeon" is just a line I am using to get rid of him. Either way, there is the inevitably awkward silence that follows the "I'm a heart surgeon" line, which then gives way to an about-face by my potential suitor.

Obviously, not all of them ran in the opposite direction. A few leaned in. A few were intrigued. Two stayed. One for nine years. The other forever. They both bought the E ticket ride that is my life. One couldn't take the high-speed turns and often diverging tracks. He threw up and left. Totally understandable. The other is still on board the Magliato coaster and is not the least bit queasy.

• • •

In life, I think we all take a practice swing. Mine was an incredible guy whom I met in my first year of medical school. He was a fourth-year medical student and had the most amazing mind I have ever encountered. I fell in love with his brain (hey, at least it wasn't his kidney), and the rest of him soon followed.

We could spend three hours at dinner engaged in nonstop interesting conversation. He was worldly, mature, and sophisticated and taught me much about life. He had such an amazing wit, and when he laughed, his whole face turned upward in a smile. It was intoxicating. Since most of my previous boyfriends were not nearly as interesting or intellectually savvy, I found him incredibly sexy. Sunday mornings were spent laboring over the *New York Times* crossword puzzle. He was (and still is) a master at it as evidenced by the fact that he does the Sunday puzzle in ink.

I met him the first day of orientation at medical school because we were paired together—he was to be my senior student adviser for the year. Instead, he became an island of love, friendship, support, and understanding in the middle of a stormy sea of library all-nighters, formaldehyde-saturated clothing, peeling the fingernails off your anatomy lab cadavers just to see what was underneath, and feeling the pain of an ulcer developing as your grades were posted for all to see. As fate would bring us together so, too, would it rip us apart. After just one terrific year together, he matched to a residency program in surgery at Case Western Reserve University in Cleveland. I would stay behind at Albany Medical College in New York. The residency match is a truly brutal process whereby you, the fourth-year medical student, list the training programs that you want to attend in rank order, and the medical/surgical programs list the potential residents that they want to train in rank order of preference. The lists go into some nebulous and frankly cruel computer that then matches up the medical students to the residency training programs based on how they ranked one another. It's like some twisted dating game similar to speed dating, which my friend Susan does. Thank God I'm not single.

After a year apart, I was finally able to get a third-year medical school spot at Case Western Reserve University School of Medicine. This was no easy feat because like getting my son into a private kindergarten in Los Angeles, there was one spot and dozens of applicants. Transferring to Cleveland meant leaving my medical school and the classmates with whom I had bonded. It also meant leaving my family, who lived only an hour away from Albany. This was probably the most difficult part of the whole deal because my family was my anchor and my support system, but this was a sacrifice I was willing to make for love. Prior to this, any boyfriend who presented an obstacle to my achieving my goal of being a surgeon was swiftly and surgically cut from my life. A big "I'm sorry" to you guys (you know who you are).

I won't lie to you: The move to Cleveland was tough on me. It took me a long time to get my bearings and establish friendships. The entire time I was there I felt like an outsider because I was joining a tight-knit group of medical students midway through the four-year program. I made this sacrifice, however, so that my boyfriend and I could be together to see if our relationship would stand the test of time. After he and I spent two years together in Ohio, it was my turn to match into a residency program in general surgery. Sacrifice number two: I ranked programs that were close to Cleveland so we could remain together during his six-year surgery subspecialty training. Ultimately, I got a spot in the general surgery program at Akron General Medical Center in Akron, Ohio. He and I spent the six years commuting to our residencies in Cleveland and Akron, respectively. When I went back into the match for my heart surgery training in 1996, after we had been together for nine years, the evil computer spit out Loyola University Med-

ical Center in Chicago. By this time, he had finished all of his
training and had a job in Cleveland. A job in which he was
quite content. He declined to leave Cleveland to go to Chicago
with me despite my pleading. I was crushed. How could he
not make this sacrifice for me? The first sacrifice that I asked
him to make. This meant that I would face two of the tough-
est years of my training alone. I remember the very first night
he left me in Chicago to return to Cleveland after he helped
me move into my apartment. I looked out over the city lights
of downtown Chicago and Navy Pier and cried for hours on
end. I didn't unpack a single item. I just sat on the floor of the
apartment feeling utterly abandoned, and sobbed. The next
morning, in a feat of strength that can only be described as
"hardened will," I picked myself up, brushed myself off, and
started my first day of residency as a cardiothoracic surgeon. I
was scared. I was lonely. But, dammit, I was determined.
Long-distance relationships are hard enough but throw in the
grueling cardiac surgery residency program and voilà! Please
exit the Magliato relationship ride to your left and watch your
step getting off.

   For the longest time I thought that I would spend the
rest of my life alone. I resigned myself to this fact. I didn't
bother with dating guys because I had a date every night for
the next two years. A date with the heart. Being a heart surgeon in training filled my life entirely. It satiated me the way
my dad's carrot mashed potatoes leave me full and in a food
coma for hours. (Incidentally, this is a mixture of carrots, potatoes, Gruyère, and cheddar cheese, and you can stand a
knife upright in the middle of a single helping of it.) Yes,
I was satisfied with my life all right until I got a taste of something different. Something sweet and lasting. Enter Nick.

"Holy s#%*! You should've f#%*^#@ seen it! I just f#%*^#@ saved this guy's f#%*^#@ life. He was f#%*^#@ dead. I mean f#%*^#@ dead as a doornail. I just split his f#%*^#@ chest open and clamped his f#%*^#@ aorta and saved his f#%*^#@ life! F#%*!" This was what Nick, the chief resident on the trauma service, heard on the other end of a phone line. I had no idea who Nick was. I was calling the trauma chief from the OR where I had just finished repairing a transected aorta on a trauma patient. The patient had been in a high-speed motor vehicle accident and the impact had torn and nearly transected his aorta. It was my first transected aorta case and I thought it was incredibly cool. I was in my second year of cardiothoracic surgery training and the attending let me do the majority of the case. I was high as a kite as I called the trauma chief, Nick, to tell him that we were bringing the patient to the ICU for him to evaluate.

Handling a patient with multiple injuries is all about triage. You find the thing that will kill him or her first and fix it first. The other injuries are then assigned a priority based on lethality. Solid organ injuries in the abdomen to the liver and spleen, for example, get priority over a fractured leg. A torn aorta or other cardiac injury goes straight to the top. One fatality in every six to ten fatal car accidents is a result of an aortic disruption. Eighty-five percent of patients with a torn or transected aorta die at the scene of the accident; 94 percent die within one hour of the injury.* A traumatic tear, similar to this but in the location of the left pulmonary vein at its junction with the heart, is what ultimately killed Princess Diana. It

*J. S. Williams et al., Aortic injury in vehicular trauma, *Annals of Thoracic Surgery* 57 (1994): 726–30.

is therefore imperative to make the diagnosis and treat it swiftly.

* * *

And so it came to be that I found myself on the phone with my future husband, letting him know that I had finished repairing the most lethal of all trauma injuries so that he could take care of the "less important" abdominal injuries. A few months passed before I had another chance to interact with the trauma chief. Again, we met over some unfortunate trauma victim with multiple injuries. How romantic! This time Nick was in the operating room with a patient who had ruptured her diaphragm (the sheet of muscle that separates the chest and abdominal cavity) during a car accident in which she was thrown from the car. Incidentally, when we were kids, my mother would never wear a seat belt because she "wanted to be thrown clear of the vehicle" during an accident, thinking that her injuries would somehow be less severe. In reality, however, 25 percent of fatal car crashes involve ejection from the vehicle. Passengers who are ejected from a car during an accident have a fatal injury rate forty times higher than those who are not thrown from the vehicle. And if you are still thinking about traveling without a seat belt, consider that your chance of a major injury of any kind increases 300 to 500 percent.

A diaphragmatic rupture can be quite a dramatic injury because the contents of your abdomen can slip through the rupture and wind up in your chest. It makes for an interesting chest X-ray that stumps medical students when they can't figure out why there are loops of bowel in the space where the lung should be. The woman had been in the car accident more than two weeks ago and her injury had been missed by the doctors at the hospital where she initially presented. This often happens with blunt diaphragm injuries because there are usually no obvious external signs of the injury. Nick had astutely made the diagnosis based on the patient's history and chest X-ray findings. He had this poor woman on the OR table and he was about to make an incision in her abdomen so that he could repair her diaphragm from below. He had instructed the on-call cardiothoracic fellow (me) to assess the patient for concomitant chest injuries. I walked into his OR, took one look at the patient's chest X-ray, and said with casual conviction, "You're doing it wrong." I then turned and abruptly left. He knew what I meant without a lengthy explanation from me that might embarrass him. There is a code of conduct among surgeons that says when you are in another surgeon's OR, you treat him or her with respect, and therefore there are ways you can address a potential error or misjudgment without making the surgeon look foolish. A raised eyebrow, a clearing of the throat, a whisper across the anesthesia drape. Announcing to the entire OR that "You're doing it wrong" was certainly pushing it, but I was two years his senior and could get away with it for now. When repairing a diaphragmatic injury that is more than a week old, it is better, in the opinion of cardiothoracic surgeons, to approach from "above"—meaning from a chest incision—because the stomach and bowel can adhere to the lungs and these adhesions must be delicately teased apart so as not to cause tears in the viscera or lung. Nick, however, was a trauma surgeon and quite adept at handling a diaphragmatic rupture from the abdomen. I was, at this juncture of my career, "hell on wheels" and adhered to a "it's my way or the highway" philosophy.

It's a wonder the man ever spoke to me after that second meeting.

But before I left the OR, I did take a moment to notice two things about this tall and slender trauma chief: (1) He had beautiful green eyes and (2) even with his surgical mask on, I could see that he had cheekbones you could park a Volkswagen on. And I made a mental note to put him on my to-do list.

A few weeks went by before I had another chance to interact with Nick. I guess three times is the charm. Our cardiothoracic surgery department was hosting a party to celebrate the retirement of one of the attending surgeons. Like Cinderella, I wouldn't be going since I was on call and couldn't leave the hospital. Not even for a few hours. One of the other cardiothoracic fellows suggested that we get one of the senior general surgery residents to cover for me so I could leave the hospital for a while. I was thrilled. This was the most social activity I had seen since I had started my fellowship more than a year earlier. I think that I was actually even more thrilled with the fact that I could go home and get a shower. Perhaps even put on clothing other than scrubs, which I had lived in all year. And, dare I think it, a little makeup? I was giddy with anticipation. One of the fellows called Nick, who generously agreed to cover for the price of a case of beer, and I dashed home to get ready.

Even though it was the late 1990s, I had permed hair and a lot of it. Why? Because it was the lowest-maintenance hairstyle around and I was a low-maintenance girl. I actually contemplated shaving my head bald during my cardiac residency but thought it would be too much work to maintain. Remember, I had no time to be a girl during these years of training.

Makeup was scarce, although I did keep one of my mother's black Maybelline eyeliner pencils by the phone to write down messages with. So getting ready consisted of hair spray and eyeliner application. Incidentally, the eyeliner pencil was so blunt from using it on paper that I nearly tore my cornea while applying it inside my lower eyelid. I found some Vaseline and used this as lip gloss. Now, what to wear? Scrubs with a belt? No. Scrubs with a scarf? No. In the recesses of my closet I had a slutty black-lace short dress from high school that I never wore . . . bingo! Off I went to the party. I had to stop by the hospital on my way to check on a patient, and while I was getting on an elevator, I briefly caught some tall guy in scrubs totally checking me out. "Creep," I thought, and hurried to the party.

The day after the party, I was in the cafeteria with two of the other cardiothoracic residents and I asked, "Have either of you talked to this Nick guy about when he wants his beer?" I was anxious about it because I was broke and needed some lead time on buying the case. As residents, we were paid fifteen thousand to twenty-five thousand dollars per year. One of the residents answered, "He's right over there, let's ask him." I turned around and there he was sitting at a table by himself. I knew it was him from the OR—cheekbones, strong jaw, green eyes. I didn't know doctors could be so cute. I said casually, "Oh, I'll go talk to him." I wandered over to where he was sitting, came up behind him so he didn't see me, leaned into his shoulder, and whispered in his right ear, "We're reneging on that case of beer and I'm taking you out instead." Ta da! First date. It worked out for him, too, since it turned out he doesn't drink beer. Sidecars are more his thing.

About a week later we both managed to find an evening

that we could be outside the hospital and he picked me up at my apartment. He greeted me at the door with "Where's the dress?" I looked at him quizzically. "You know," he said, "the one you wore at the hospital the other night." "Oh, you're the creep!" I replied. That was my opening line on our first date.

We went to dinner at the Cheesecake Factory on the lower level of the Hancock Building on Michigan Avenue. It was the best first date ever. We spent the night talking about our families and our lives. For the first time, I was around someone who had a similar upbringing to mine. The similarities were incredible and I felt instantly at ease with Nick. He grew up as a PK— a pastor's kid. His father was a Lutheran minister who preached mainly at the local prison, and his mother was a teacher and later a homemaker. He had six siblings, one of whom died in early childhood from congenital heart disease. They grew up with very little. They burned firewood to heat their home in the small town of Askov, Minnesota. They farmed their land. They got their clothes from Goodwill. Like me, he was the only medical doctor in the family. I left the date thinking that he could be my soul mate.

We dated for the remaining time that we were at Loyola Medical Center. It wasn't easy to find time to spend together so we found other ways to express our love. We would leave love notes written on the back of our cafeteria food coupons in each other's white-coat pockets, which hung on a hook outside the OR. When I finished a case, I knew that I would have a note secretly placed in my coat waiting for me and so did he. We had a secret page number that we would send into each other's pagers that meant "I'm thinking about you" when one of us received it. Every morning, whichever one of us didn't spend the night in the hospital would go to Dunkin' Donuts and get the other person's favorite coffee, write a note on the Styrofoam cup, and leave it stashed in a secret location in the surgical ICU to retrieve and take on rounds. Mine was always a medium vanilla, black. His was a medium, regular, light and sweet.

We somehow found a balance between the rigors of our jobs and finding the time to put into nourishing our relationship. There was no room for pressure or stress in our relationship because we each had our fill of that in our jobs. Our relationship blossomed just as fellowships were looming in the distance for both of us. I wanted to spend another year of training beyond my cardiothoracic residency in a transplant fellowship and Nick wanted to spend a fellowship year in surgical critical care following his general surgery residency. The two best heart/lung transplant fellowships in the country were at the University of Pittsburgh Medical Center and Stanford University Hospital. These were the only two programs to which I applied. If I was going to endure another year of training, then I wanted the best. Nick had several outstanding programs to choose from for his fellowship and one of them happened to be at Pittsburgh. It felt like déjà vu. Would he choose Pittsburgh so we could be together or would he leave me to pursue a different fellowship location? I didn't pressure him. I gave him the space he needed to make his choice. I let fate take over.

He chose Pittsburgh and the year together strengthened our relationship. Our fellowships demanded a lot from us, but we managed to find time to enjoy life together. In the middle of the year, Nick received an unexpected call from the chief of the liver transplant program at the UCLA Medical Center in Los Angeles. UCLA was one of the most prestigious liver transplant programs in the world, and its chairman, Dr. Ronald W. Busuttil, was a maverick in liver transplantation. He had heard about Nick at a liver conference he had attended and wanted to personally invite him to do a two-year fellowship in liver transplant surgery at UCLA. Dr. Busuttil handpicks his fellows from around the country and this was quite an unexpected honor for Nick. As fate would have it, a nearby medical center in Los Angeles was also looking for a heart transplant surgeon. Amazing things occur if you just have a little faith that things will work out for the best.

When we arrived together in LA, we asked someone, "How do you get to the ocean?" and they told us to just drive to the end of Sunset Boulevard. So we did. And in the process we found a place to live where we could see the ocean every day. Not bad for two kids from Minnesota and New York.

We got engaged on the beach at the stroke of midnight at the millennium and were married two years later. When two people get married, there comes a moment when you just have to take that last leap of faith that you are doing the right thing. That moment can come at any time. For some it comes well before the wedding; for others it comes while you are actually at the altar. The most senior heart surgeon by age and experience with whom I have ever worked used to say in the OR, "Feel the force." It is, of course, taken from the Jedi Knights of Star Wars fame. He said this whenever there was a moment in surgery when your sense of sight or touch might misguide you in some way. An example would be when you are trying to get an umbilical tape (named because it was originally used to tie off the umbilici of calves and foals) safely around the aorta and you can neither see nor feel the backside of this, the largest blood vessel connected to the heart. A wrong move could result in a potentially lethal puncture of the aorta at the most posterior aspect. Repairing a puncture like this would be extremely difficult. And so, as he said, you need to "feel the force" and rely on an intangible sense that every surgeon has but few surgeons may be truly in touch with. "Feeling the force" is what you must do when you make that final commitment to marriage. Forget about your known senses and rely on the force that you feel when you are around that person. Find that safe plane that connects the two of you.

We finally felt that force in our lives together and were married a year later in a quiet little Lutheran church in Venice, California. It was just the two of us and God. No big wedding. No family. No reception. The wedding was about us and our commitment to each other with no distractions. Nick was supposed to be in charge of the music, but when I entered the church I noticed the distinct absence of any musicians. I assumed that he was probably too busy in the weeks before the wedding and simply forgot. As I began to walk down the aisle, I heard, faintly at first and then unmistakably, a lone bagpiper playing outside the church at a distance. Bagpipes have a very special meaning to me because like my sister and father before me, I graduated from college to a bagpipe procession, which is a longstanding tradition at Union College. Nick hadn't forgotten the music and, in fact, had reached out and embraced one of my fondest memories of accomplishment to make our wedding special to me.

Nick knows me. He knows the most intimate details of my life. He knows the quiet recesses of my heart. I guess I wasn't fair when I said that my personal relationships with men other than my colleagues have been the most difficult to sustain. After all, it takes just one. One that will last forever.

10

We've Come a Long Way, Baby

An ounce of prevention is worth a pound of cure.

—Benjamin Franklin

Donna lay awake at night with the fear that if she closed her eyes, she would not awaken in the morning. Such is the apprehension that comes with the knowledge that your heart is diseased.

As she lay in her bed, her fingers slowly moved across her chest. She felt the flatness of her breastbone, but as she neared its midline she felt a small ridge. Almost imperceptible at first, but then, yes, she could discern a definite hill in what is normally supposed to be flat terrain.

She moved her fingers up the slope of this fleshy incline and reached its pinnacle, where a rough seam was present. She felt a sudden break in the softly textured smoothness of her body. Like running your hand along a fine suede cushion and coming to a line of stitching, it ruins the tactile moment and you wonder, "Why would someone put a seam here that alters the rich flow of the fabric?" It seems careless and abnormal.

When Donna opens her eyes, however, the ridge and its

rough peak are gone. She must have dozed off for, in reality, Donna's chest is unmarred. She has been a survivor of heart disease since 1979. Back then, we didn't operate on women. We put them on bed rest, treated their "anxiety attack," and gave them aspirin. Donna is a survivor not because of her medical treatment but because, unlike Dorothy, she didn't ignore her symptoms. Donna understood and, therefore, was able to modify her risk factors.

On a warm July morning in 1979 Donna went running, as was her routine. She was thirty-five years old. She was a movie producer at the top of her game. By lunch she didn't "feel so good." She was cold and clammy and her usually crisp white Armani blouse was sticking to her skin. She made it through her "power lunch" but went home to rest. By 4:00 p.m. she was lying on her bathroom floor pressing her forehead against the marble tile because its coolness made her feel better. Ironically, on her way home, she had stopped at the home of her internist, who was a personal friend. She told him that she felt generally unwell and had an awful pain in her chest that seemed like it was "boring a hole clean through" to her back. He told her that she had a "diaphragmatic stitch" in her side from running that morning. (Now, incidentally, would be a good time to tell you that in a survey done a mere four years ago, fewer than one in five physicians recognized that more women die of heart disease than men each year, and among primary care physicians, only 8 percent knew this fact.*

*Lori Mosca, MD, et al., "Women's heart risk underestimated by doctors, resulting in less preventative care than men," *Circulation* NR05-1011. February 1, 2004.

But Donna knew something was wrong. Very wrong. We all have a built-in sixth sense about our bodies. We just need to trust it. We are the nurturers. We are the caregivers. We are the mommies, the aunts, the grandmothers, the sisters. We care for those around us and we do not listen to our own bodies when they cry out for healing and attention. "I'll deal with it later" is the mantra of most women when confronted by their own health issues, and yet we are the first ones to put our dads on a train to Memorial Sloan-Kettering to have their prostate radiated. Ladies, it's time to put *your* health issues at the head of the queue.

So what did Donna do? She brought herself straight to the hospital. She didn't care if when she got there they would just dismiss her with a "stomach flu." She cared more about her survival than she did about the possible embarrassment of going to the hospital for something that might be non–life threatening. A good lesson for us all. I have had so many women tell me that they did not go to the ER when they experienced chest pain because of their concern that it might be a false alarm. So what? You waste an afternoon in the ER. At least you are alive to go home in time for dinner.

The tests eventually showed that Donna had had a heart attack. She was admitted to the coronary care unit and was treated with the medications available at the time and bed rest. Sure, at night she finds it difficult to sleep because she worries about her heart, but today she is alive. She is beautiful. She is my friend. And she is unscathed by heart disease.

"We've come a long way, baby" was the slogan for the Virginia Slims advertisement featuring the 1970s supermodel Cheryl Tiegs. In the print ad she is beautiful and svelte, confidently wearing a pants suit and smoking a cigarette. Certainly cigarettes can be glamorous and can make you look hip—or cool. But how glamorous is it to have a toe tag? Really. And so I beg to differ with Virginia Slims. When today, at this very moment, heart disease is still the number one killer of women, we haven't really come a long way, baby—at all!

What saved Donna's life? Pure and simple, it was knowledge. Of all the things that women can do to avoid heart disease—quit smoking, exercise, diet—knowledge is the most important. We have done such an incredible job with breast cancer awareness that through educating the female public, women know the risk factors for breast cancer, the signs of breast cancer, how to do self-exams and regularly engage in screening mammograms. Because of this awareness campaign and knowledge, women are diagnosed at an earlier stage and survive breast cancer. Now, if we could just launch the same awareness campaign for cardiovascular disease, we would affect women's survival in numbers that would be unprecedented.

When I lecture to women about heart disease, I always leave them with two things to remember. I tell them that if they just employ these two measures, they will be able to stay away from me, the chest-cracker. Now, I'm a nice gal and generally fun to be around, but you don't want to be on the receiving end of my scalpel. Trust me. The two things are these: (1) Know your numbers and (2) know your symptoms. I want this to be your mantra, like "Save the cheerleader, save the world," for all of you *Heroes* fans out there. What I mean by this is know your heart health numbers—your total cholesterol, your "good" cholesterol (HDL), your "bad" cholesterol (LDL), your triglycerides, your blood pressure, and if you are a diabetic, your blood sugar. Why? Because if you know these numbers, you will own these numbers and strive to keep them in the normal range. Too many women walk around not knowing their numbers, so they have no idea that they are at risk of dying from heart disease. Ahhhhhhhh. Ignorance is bliss. That is, until your family finds you dead on your kitchen floor.

Case in point: My older sister called me the other day to tell me that she just got back from her gynecologist's office and has good news. "Everything is great, Kath, my internal exam was normal, my Pap smear came back normal, my cholesterol was two seventy-seven, and I don't need to go back to the doctor for a year so I'm just on my way over to Friendly's for a Reese's Pieces sundae to celebrate." Now, I feel sorry for her, really I do. After all, it's got to be hard having a sister who is a heart surgeon. So I say to her, "Nancy, can you back up to the part about your cholesterol?" "Well," she answers, "it's two seventy-seven but that's no big deal, right? He [her doctor] didn't really say much about that and my Pap smear's okay." "Nancy," I say, trying to be reasonably delicate about this, "can you do me a favor? Go into the garage, get a shovel, and dig a hole for yourself in the backyard." Like I said, it's a bitch to have a sister who's a heart surgeon. The lesson here is that if my own sister can blissfully walk around with a cholesterol level of 277 milligrams / deciliters (mg/dl), then anyone can.

So what kind of numbers do we want to see? Not 277 mg/dl, I can assure you. We want to see your total cholesterol under 200 mg/dl. The general rule of thumb is 100 plus your age. It is, however, amazing to me that 58 percent of women have a cholesterol greater than 200 mg/dl and 28 percent of women have a cholesterol greater than 240 mg/dl. We want your HDL to be greater than 60 mg/dl and your LDL less than 160 mg/dl if you have fewer than two risk factors for heart disease, less than 130 mg/dl if you have more than two risk factors, and less than 100 mg/dl if you have known heart disease. Your triglyceride goal should be less than 150 mg/dl. It used to be that for blood pressure, we would accept a level of 140/80 millimeters of mercury (mmHg). More recent research has told us that this is not an acceptable blood pressure. This number is considered "hypertension" and greatly increases your risk for heart disease. We want your blood pressure closer to 120/80 mmHg. I have a babysitter who is in her early thirties. She is bright and very mature for her age. She works out regularly and spends all day running after my boys. She eats well except for the occasional sweet, which is her only vice. To look at her, you would never think that her blood pressure runs greater than 140/80 mmHg. Although my husband and I repeatedly caution her to get her blood pressure under better control, she blows it off, as any thirty-year-old would. She's young and otherwise healthy. Why bother? Because even at such a young age, *especially* at a young age, hypertension can cause heart damage, which will manifest itself later in life. But women who are young feel invincible and aren't really concerned about their health.

For diabetics it's worse. It is estimated that 18.2 million people have diabetes and nearly one-third are unaware that they have this disease. A simple blood test called hemoglobin A1c or a fasting blood sugar can diagnose it. For women it's a double whammy because if you are a woman with diabetes, you have a higher relative risk for heart disease than a man with diabetes. Therefore, it is imperative for a diabetic woman to know her blood sugar and keep it under strict control.

The two other risk factors for cardiovascular disease that

you need to know are smoking and obesity. I shouldn't have to even mention these to you because everyone knows that smoking is bad and obesity is worse. You probably know, for example, that smoking increases your risk for heart disease two to six times more than that of a nonsmoker. But did you know that passive smokers who inhale smoke inadvertently from a nearby smoker have a 30 percent increase risk of heart attack? Did you also know that a woman who smokes and takes oral contraceptives increases her risk for heart disease by 20 percent? This is a major contributing factor to why we are seeing young women in their thirties with cardiovascular illness.

Obesity is an epidemic among children, adolescents, and adults. It is responsible for all of the following cardiovascular-related illnesses: heart attack, angina, heart failure, sudden death, abnormal heart rhythm, high blood pressure, metabolic syndrome, diabetes, abnormal lipid levels, peripheral vascular disease, and stroke. Because of this one single risk factor and its impact on cardiovascular illness, the current generation of children will be the first not to outlive the generation before them.

So what about Donna? She didn't have high cholesterol or diabetes and her blood pressure was normal. She didn't smoke nor was she obese. There are, unfortunately, two risk factors for heart disease that we can do nothing about: family history and age. Although at times you may want to disown your family, you can never disown your own genes. Donna had a family history of heart disease from which she couldn't escape. For a family history to "count," it has to be a first-degree relative (mother, father, brother, sister) who has had cardiovascular disease (heart disease, hypertension, stroke). If it is a female relative who has had cardiovascular disease, then her disease has to have occurred before the age of sixty-five and for a male relative it has to be before the age of fifty-five. So, for example, your grandmother who had heart disease at the age of seventy wouldn't count as a family risk factor but your sister with heart disease at the age of sixty-three would.

As for age, you can have all the plastic surgery in the world and may look twenty-five on the outside, but ladies, if you are fifty-five years of age or older, you automatically have a risk factor that you can't escape. It is a sad, ironic truth that many women who undergo plastic surgery procedures after age fifty-five are not screened for heart disease preoperatively. An ironic truth that can be lethal.

And so remember, ladies, I implore you to understand the risk factors for heart disease and to know your numbers. I want you to be able to rattle these numbers off the same way that you can rattle off your Social Security number. It can save your life.

As for the second part of this mantra, "Know your symptoms," I will let Cristin, who arrived at my hospital DOA, tell you about that. You'll be meeting her shortly . . .

11

Dead on Arrival

RECEIVED AN E-MAIL A FEW MONTHS AGO FROM MY friend Ann, who just happens to be the best damn cardiologist I have ever had the honor to work with. Together, she and I spent some all-nighters at the bedsides of patients we were trying to keep alive. We were a good team. Maybe even a great one. I was glad to get her e-mail because I hadn't heard from her in a while. Ann had quit the rat race of chasing down heart disease and treating it with medication. She retired to a farm in her hometown with a pretty red barn with solar panels on the roof and a room for her to dabble in arts and crafts. She also keeps a little cabin in the woods that is hidden deeply among the sleeping sequoia giants. Ann, for the first time in a long time, is quite content. It wasn't that she burned out—she was a superstar and loved to take care of patients. The sicker they were, the brighter she shined. I think it was that she just hit the glass ceiling of medicine so hard she got a concussion. That, and a desire to spend more time with her mom. I've done that, too, you know. I've cracked my head on the same glass ceiling so many times that I've lost count. Thankfully, I have thick skull—*testa dura,* they say in Italian. I guess I get it from my dad.

In her e-mail, she told me that Mended Hearts wanted me to speak at one of their chapter meetings in Anaheim. As it turns out, the Anaheim chapter president is a former patient of ours whom she and I took care of during his heart transplant seven years ago. I remember his transplant well and can vouch for the fact that this lovely man is as beautiful on the inside as he is on the outside.

Mended Hearts is a national nonprofit organization that was started by a heart surgeon, Dwight Harken, in 1951 when he brought together four patients whom he had operated on to form a support group. Through their common experience of having had heart surgery, they provided "compassion, hope and encouragement" (their mission statement) to other postoperative patients. Today, there are thousands of members who dedicate their time to giving back to other patients through hospital visits, support group meetings, and hosting educational seminars. According to their website, they make approximately 227,000 visits to hospitalized patients and 30,000 visits to family members yearly. I was honored to be asked to speak at a chapter meeting.

Because you can throw a stone from Anaheim Memorial Medical Center to Disneyland, I brought my kids and their caretaker with me and dropped them off at the the Happiest Place on Earth. When my lecture concluded, it was almost 4:00 p.m. and I knew that getting on the I-5 freeway and back to the hospital at that hour was futile. Traffic in LA is just an unavoidable part of life—like death and taxes. So I headed over to Disneyland to join Nicholas and Gabriel. How great it is to work and be a mommy all in the same day!

We hit several rides in Adventure and then went to Frontierland to take the Pirates of the Caribbean ride—the kids' favorite. (Thank God they had already done the Flying Dumbo ride—shortest ride in the park, longest line.) Pirates of the Caribbean turned out to be a great ride—it was air-conditioned (a bonus in the Anaheim summer heat), had some exciting dips and turns, and you to got to see Johnny Depp. There were several signs during the ride that read DEAD MEN TELL NO TALES. And while this may be true, dead women *do* tell tales . . .

• • •

The second time I met Cristin she was naked on a cold steel slab in the hospital morgue. A four-by-four-inch block of wood was under her head to keep it propped up. Propping up the head in this manner makes it easier to saw open the skull circumferentially to allow a full examination of the brain. While I was standing next to her waiting for the autopsy to start, a pathology lab assistant, without warning, pulled the block of wood out from under her head. Her head quickly dropped back and hit the table with a loud hollow *clang!* It was as if someone had dropped a cantaloupe on a stainless steel kitchen counter. The impact of her head on the table made me flinch because I momentarily had forgotten that she wasn't alive.

Dead patients can tell their tale through an autopsy. We learn about their life and their death. Did they have children? Did they eat well? Did they smoke? Did they have cosmetic surgery that they never told anyone about? In an autopsy, every medical detail is revealed. We learn so much from a post-mortem examination. It is such a shame that health insurance companies will no longer pay for this, the final surgical procedure. If not paid for by the hospital, the financial burden of an autopsy is placed upon the family of the deceased. At a cost of two thousand to four thousand dollars per autopsy, fewer and fewer are being done, and so fewer dead men and women are able to tell their tales.

I have made it a point to attend the autopsy of every patient I have come in contact with, whether just to render a consultation or to perform surgery. It is the last gesture of respect that you can pay to your patient. Pathologists are the true astronauts of the medical universe. They explore the deep space of the human body both on a macroscopic and microscopic level. They leave no gallstone unturned. No body cavity is off-limits. They are fearless in their surgical dissection because there is no life to preserve, only the postmortem memory of that life. One of my best college buddies went into pathology and forensic medicine. He had the most inquisitive and probing mind and the gentlest nature—the traits of a good pathologist.

My first autopsy of sorts was in medical school during my anatomy course. Four students team up and each group gets a body that was generously donated for this purpose. I am so grateful to the woman who donated her body to our team. If you asked me, "Of all the professors, medical doctors, surgeons, fellows, residents, and nurses who taught you, from whom did you learn the most?" I would say without hesitation that it was the anonymous woman who willingly gave me her body to dissect. Each team named its cadaver. We called ours Abra as in "abra cadaver." This may seem disrespectful, but please understand that we needed to impose an ounce of levity on what we were doing each day.

The anatomy course, given in the first year of medical school, was the course that every medical student eagerly anticipated. The anticipation, however, was peppered with apprehension and a little fear thrown in for good measure. Just entering the anatomy lab was a daunting task. When you walked through the threshold, there were rows and rows of tables upon which lay thick black plastic body bags smudged and shiny with the grease of the cadaver's adipose tissue. This body fat grease was particularly annoying because it got all over everything and was impossible to wipe off, like smeared butter on a pair of eyeglasses. Neurologists say that the olfactory sense imprints the strongest memories in your brain. More so than sight, sound, taste, or touch. I can close my eyes right now and still feel and smell the sting of formaldehyde in my nostrils and sinuses. It's sharp. Acrid. It burns like smelling salts. It's also an inescapable smell that permeates everything—your clothes, your books, your skin, your eyebrows. Everyone at school knew who was "doing anatomy" by their reek.

I spent hours in that anatomy lab dissecting such structures as the seven branches of the facial nerve—one of the most difficult and intricate dissections. Take the pad of your right thumb and touch it to the angle of your jaw below your earlobe on the right side of your face and let the palm and fingers of your right hand splay out across your cheek and face. That's where the facial nerve and its branches run. The nerve is so fragile and delicate that dissecting it from within the facial muscle and parotid gland is like trying to dissect a spider's wed embedded in Play-Doh. You must painstakingly tease it out while trying not to injure any of its wispy branches.

Mostly, I worked at night. Since the lab was open twenty-four hours a day, we had unlimited access to our bodies. You could tell who the real "gunners" were because we'd be up there in the lab probing, dissecting, memorizing into the wee hours. I have to tell you, it was a little scary to be there at night, but I liked the quiet. Not completely quiet, however. The hum of the fluorescent lights overhead was my constant acoustic companion. Picture in your mind the scene from the 1978 movie *Coma* (directed by Michael Crichton) when Geneviève Bujold walks into the room in the Jefferson Institution where all of the comatose patients are hanging suspended from the ceiling by cables embedded in their bones. The anatomy lab had that same sense of serenity and horror.

But I digress from Cristin's story. Recall that the morgue is the second time that I met Cristin. The first time was in the ER, where she arrived in full cardiac arrest from a treadmill at the local gym. She was thirty-five years old—nearly a decade younger than me. Blond and beautiful. She had a killer bod. Lean, fit, with breasts that couldn't possibly be real (they were).

I didn't treat Cristin. There was no need. She was already dead. I was in the ER to see another woman who was having a heart attack when I just happened to walk past the trauma bay—a large, surgically equipped ER facility reserved exclusively for patients with potentially lethal injuries, such as gunshot wounds, stab wounds, high-speed motor vehicle accidents, full cardiac arrests. Every high-volume ER has one. As I walked past, I noticed this very young, very beautiful woman lying on a gurney. I thought, at first, that she was asleep, which I thought was odd. As I got a fuller view of her, I saw the telltale sign that she was not alive—an endotracheal tube was sticking out of her mouth, not connected to anything. Not to a ventilator. Not to an ambu bag. Not even to oxygen. The trauma bay was in complete disarray—a sign that the ER doctors had put up a good fight. Four-by-four-inch sponges, syringes, needles, IV bags and tubing, discarded "amps" (ampules) of sodium "bicarb" (bicarbonate) were everywhere. No blood, though. Her blue yoga pants with an energetic paisley pattern had been cut away from ankle to hip in the crude way that only heavy serrated scissors, or trauma shears, can cut. Her matching sky-blue sports bra was also cut away, revealing rectangular burns with rounded edges on her chest. The macabre tattoo, if you will, imprinted upon her flesh by an external defibrillator.

If Cristin could tell her tale, it would go something like this:

I'm a health nut. I eat only natural organic raw foods and I use only holistic remedies to treat illness. I think I am really in touch with my body. I exercise every day and practice yoga for relaxation. My only vice is that I watch TV, mostly the History Channel and the Discovery Channel. I love medical shows, though, like House, Grey's Anatomy, and ER. A week before I died I had a toothache in my lower molars. I treated it with topical clove oil and white willow bark, which I got at Whole Foods, and this seemed to help a little. But the pain in my jaw kept nagging me, so I reluctantly went to a dentist. He pulled one tooth, which didn't help, and so he pulled another . . . and another. This seemed like a completely unnatural treatment to me, so I just stopped going back to the dentist. How was I to know that jaw pain is a symptom of heart disease? The medical shows that I watch on TV all show heart attacks as crushing pain at the center of your chest with the actor sweating, red-faced, and short of breath. The heart attack victim clutches his chest and falls to the ground, where he lapses into unconsciousness. It's very

dramatic. Look, other than having a little heart disease in
my family, I have no other risk factors. I mean, just
LOOK AT ME. I'm young, I'm fit and healthy, I'm
dead . . . I'm dead . . . I'm . . .

We've been sold a bill of goods by the media that says that this is what heart disease looks like. That may be true— for men. Women have much more subtle symptoms. Half of women have no chest pain at all! Other symptoms of heart disease that are unique to women include jaw pain (like Cristin's), arm pain, mild shortness of breath, indigestion or "heartburn," and nausea. The most common symptom that women get is fatigue. Fatigue! What woman isn't fatigued from multitasking and dual role-playing trying to balance career and family? And what do you think is the most common way that women present with heart disease? *Dead!* In more than 50 percent of women, this is the first symptom of heart disease. They just show up dead in my ER.

We are the mommies. We are the nurturers. But we are too busy taking care of everyone else around us and we forget to take care of ourselves. We need to listen to what our bodies are telling us, for they do tell tales. Cristin wishes she had.

12

Jackson Pollock

MY FRIEND TIM OWNS TWO ORIGINAL JACKSON POL-locks. I have been a fan of Pollock's work since I stood in front of *No. 5, 1948*, on loan to the Louvre. To me, Pollock's paintings are about beauty and chaos. Two words that I believe sum up my life in its entirety. When you stand within inches of a Jackson Pollock, all you can see are strands of chaotic paint. When you move away from the piece and give it a respectful distance, you see its beauty, and a sense of serenity begins to form within the painting. I suppose when I look closely at the details of my life I see nothing but chaos, but when I step back and look at my life, counting all of my blessings, I see beauty. Pure, simple beauty.

• • •

Jackson Pollock, was what I thought as I rounded the corner of the ICU in a full sprint. I heard one of my partners yell "KATHY! WAIT!" somewhere behind me, but I was several lengths ahead of him, having outdistanced him from the parking lot, and was not about to wait. The only time I had slowed down was when I hit the elevator (the stairwell was closed; otherwise, I would have taken that). I traveled the six floors to the ICU doubled over, hands on my knees, trying to catch my breath, which came in short, irregular gasps. I know I need to take more spinning classes, I just don't have the time.

When I turned the corner and finally made it to Rosie's bedside, there were streaks of blood splattered on all four walls in a pattern not unlike a Pollock. Some strands of blood were thick, others quite delicate and wispy. They were all in various states of drying, which gave them each a different hue of red. Blood darkens as it dries until it reaches an almost black coloration. Chaos was everywhere.

I was a young attending surgeon and lived twenty-five minutes from the hospital because I could not afford to live any closer. One of my other partners who lives closest to the hospital was already in the process of "cracking her chest," the procedure whereby we rapidly open a patient's chest at the bedside. It is called cracking the chest because when we remove the sternal wires embedded in the breastbone during the chest closure, the chest simply springs apart like when you crack open a ripe summer watermelon to reveal its fleshy pulp. This procedure is usually done for profound and uncontrollable bleeding, which is what happened in Rosie's case.

Rosie had had mitral valve surgery by a senior surgeon a few days earlier because she had a "leaky" valve. The mitral valve is so named because it is shaped like a mitre—the liturgical headdress worn by bishops or abbots. It is one of the four valves in your heart that regulate blood flow through each of the four chambers. It is located between the atrium (upper chamber) and ventricle (lower chamber) on the left side of your heart. The heart's valves open and close forty million times per year or approximately two billion times in the average life span. With time and certain disease processes, such as rheumatic fever, any of your four valves can fail to function properly. When a valve is narrowed by the buildup of calcium on its leaflets, it can become tight in a process known as stenosis. Blood is inhibited from passing easily in a forward direction from chamber to chamber. When the shape of the leaflets of the valve or their proximity to each other becomes distorted, the leaflets don't coapt, or come together properly, to close the valve. This causes the valve to leak and is called regurgitation. Blood is allowed to flow backward between the chambers of the heart. In Rosie's case, she had severe mitral valve regurgitation.

When the valves in your heart fail owing either to regurgitation or stenosis, it puts a tremendous strain on your heart. As a consequence, the chambers in your heart become thickened and/or dilate and the heart's ability to pump blood is diminished. This leads to heart failure. It is therefore imperative that we either repair or replace the faulty valve. Between 71,000 and 79,000 heart valve replacements are done each year in the United States, and 265,000 implants are performed annually worldwide. If we replace your valve, we can put in one of two types: a tissue or biological valve or a mechanical valve. A tissue valve is either made from a pig valve or fashioned from the sac around the heart of a cow (bovine pericardial valve). We can also use a valve taken from a dead person (a homograft) or borrow the pulmonary valve from the right side of your heart (autograft). The advantage of having a tissue valve is that you do not need to take lifelong anticoagulation medication or blood thinners such as Couma-din. The disadvantage is that it will last approximately twenty years, with 30 percent needing to be replaced in ten years and 50 percent needing replacement within fifteen years. A mechanical valve is made from metals and materials such as titanium, graphite, pyrolytic carbon, and polyester. Mechanical valves require that you take a blood thinner for the rest of your life. The advantage of a mechanical valve, though, is that it will last your lifetime.

Rosie's mitral valve had suffered irreparable damage and had to be replaced. We chose to implant a mechanical valve because she was young and beyond childbearing years. Normally, we allow patients to make the choice as to which type valve they would prefer, but Rosie hadn't been diagnosed with valve disease until the point at which she became so short of breath that she had to be sedated and intubated within minutes of arriving at our ER. We brought her, unconscious and on a ventilator, to the operating room and made her choices for her.

She had been to a doctor—two, in fact. She had been having progressive shortness of breath for several weeks. The first doctor, an internist, diagnosed her with asthma and gave her inhalers. The second doctor, a pulmonologist (a specialist in lung disease), diagnosed her with the flu, because in addition to the shortness of breath, she had become run-down and fatigued. He gave her antibiotics. This is an all-too-common scenario for women—they are dismissed by a doctor without further testing for symptoms that could be related to heart disease. Case in point: A 1999 *New England Journal of Medicine* article by Kevin A. Schulman, MD, and colleagues reported a Georgetown University study that was done to test whether or not there is a bias against women with heart disease based on gender difference alone. In this study, 720 primary care physicians were shown a videotape of actors and actresses in a hospital setting acting out the classic symptoms of heart disease. The physicians were then asked which "patient" most likely had heart disease and should be referred for further testing. One hundred percent of the actors were referred for more in-depth diagnostic testing and only 60 percent of the actresses were referred, even though they portrayed identical symptoms!

For Rosie, however, despite a relatively swift diagnosis in the ER and a successful lifesaving operation, something had cut loose in her chest. Three hours earlier during rounds she had been sitting up in a chair eating breakfast. I had debated removing her chest tubes because they were no longer draining blood. We normally remove these within twenty-four to forty-eight hours of surgery. I decided to leave them in for another day. This turned out to be a very fortunate decision, because when she did bleed, the nurses diagnosed it immediately. They saw the telltale sign of blood suddenly pouring out of both tubes simultaneously and filling the collection chamber known as a Pleur-evac.

It was a fluke. A horrible, horrible fluke. Rosie had a violent coughing fit and just suddenly started bleeding. I cannot explain why things like this happen. I have altogether stopped trying because it rattles my faith to try to find some reasonable explanation. Like trying to understand why the recent earthquake in China occurred or why the 2004 Indian Ocean tsunami happened. It defies logic. All I know are the facts: One minute I was hiking in the tranquillity of Temescal Canyon with my husband and sons and the next minute I was tearing Rosie's chest open.

We have a special cart in our ICU called the cracking-the-chest cart. Although this nomenclature lacks imagination, I am at a loss to think of many good alternative titles. The "let's undo all of my fine work" cart or the "give me every damn surgical instrument available right away" cart doesn't really cut it either. Essentially, this cart is filled with drawers that contain every possible item that we need to open a patient's chest at the bedside—scalpels, scissors, hemostats, forceps, sterile drapes, gowns, gloves, masks, surgical caps, gauze, suture, syringes, needles, and so forth. Each drawer is clearly labeled so that in the fray of things we can find exactly what we need. We go to great lengths to make sure that the cart is well stocked and that everything is in its place. If I open the "wire-cutter" drawer and find cotton swabs, I swear I will lose it right then and there. That is why no one—*no one*—ever touches that cart except the cardiothoracic surgeons. No doctor or nurse ever "borrows" something from that cart because it is easier than having to walk all the way to central supply in the basement, for fear of losing a limb as a consequence.

The drawer I hate most is the bottom drawer. Aptly positioned because it is the last drawer we open when we crack a chest. This drawer has no label. It doesn't need one. We all know what's in it—sternal wires and a few packs of large-caliber No. 1 suture, which we use for chest closure. If the drawer did have a label, it would read DEATH or YOU TRIED AND FAILED. But who on earth would put a label like that on a cart filled with supplies that are supposed to save a life?

The cart is rectangular in shape and measures, in centimeters, 87 h × 67 w × 46 d. It is on wheels so that we can quickly move it to any bedside in the hospital, but it is always docked in the cardiac surgical ICU. On the top of the cart sits an enormous tray of surgical instruments. It is called—what else?—the cracking-the-chest tray. Again, no imagination. The tray is covered with a bright blue paper wrapping that signifies the contents have been sterilized. Sterile pale yellow tape is crisscrossed on the top of the blue wrapping—one horizontal ribbon of tape running from side to side and one vertical ribbon running from top to bottom. At first glance, it looks like a well-wrapped present, but like fruitcake, this is one present that you never want to be on the receiving end of.

The tray contains an overabundant number of surgical instruments. As if we were climbing K2, we want to have every possible item we need so we can address any crisis that we face during a bedside chest exploration. For once you are halfway into someone's chest—halfway to the K2 summit—there is no turning back to get something you need and forgot to bring along in your pack. Of course, this does present some problems as well—it makes it very hard to find the exact Castroviejo needle holder or DeBakey forceps with the fine tip that you need among the rubble of instruments in the tray. This sends you digging into the pile of stainless steel, tungsten carbide, and titanium, disrupting the order of everything on the tray. The shuffling of the instruments makes a sound not unlike rummaging in your silverware drawer looking for that special oyster shell caviar spoon or that favorite pearl-handled butter knife. Digging. Digging. Digging for what you need, your gloved hand slick with blood sliding among the glistening steel hoping to find that sixty-degree-angled Potts scissors that you simply must have. Now! All while someone is dying two feet away from you.

I have taken it upon myself, recently, to revise the cracking-the-chest tray in an attempt to make it less confusing and more user-friendly. When all is said and done, we really only need six immediate items to open the chest, and so I designed a separate, smaller tray to house these critical instruments. I call the tray the open-first tray. I could have gotten fancy and called it the primo tray or the what-you-absolutely-positively-need tray, but I guess that I have fallen prey to a lack of imagination.

The six items that you need in order of use are:

1. *No. 10 blade scalpel*
2. *Large Mayo scissors*
3. *Wire holders*
4. *Wire cutters*
5. *Chest spreader/retractor*
6. *Suction catheter*
7. *Your index finger*

As one can clearly see, I have added a seventh item, your index finger, to hold pressure over the bleeding site if you are lucky enough to find it. In Rosie's case, I needed three fingers to cover the tear in her right atrium. Even three fingers, at times, could not adequately dam the flood of blood that poured out of her heart with each beat. To get a better purchase on the bleeding site, I had to get up on the bed with her. I knelt next to her with both of my knees resting against her upper-left arm, which hung lifelessly at her side. I stabilized myself by keeping my quadriceps taut and bracing my right arm, elbow locked, next to her left ear. With my left hand covering the hole in her heart, I formed a human tripod, balancing most of my weight on my legs—a position usually reserved for a game of Twister with my kids. I remained frozen in this position for the next thirty minutes. If

I moved a fractional amount or shifted my weight in any limb, my left hand would move ever so slightly and a torrent of blood would expel from her heart.

The worst of this was not the burning pain in my thighs from lactic acid buildup, nor the bony ache that crept into the joint of my elbow from being locked in a hyperextended position, nor the numbness that overcame all five fingers of my left hand, which had now become one with her right atrium. The worst part was the blood that managed to seep through my fingers with each beat. Red blood cells are only 6.6 to 7.5 microns in diameter and these tiny spheres inevitably found their way through the interstices between my fingers no matter how tightly I held them together. The blood was initially warm as it passed over my fingers. Bathwater warm. Body-temperature warm. But soon it ran cold. As if someone had plucked it from the top shelf of my refrigerator next to the almond milk that I now have to serve my children because every other milk has hormones in it.

Why did Rosie's blood run cold? Because she had no more blood. The blood she was born with was all gone. The average seventy-kilogram (154-pound) person has 5.2 liters (5.5 quarts) of blood and we had spent all of it. Like putting your life savings into a Top Dollar slot machine at the Bellagio, we had spent it all. Quickly. Without knowing it. Without keeping track of our losses. The cold blood running through my fingers was, in fact, banked blood, which came refrigerated from the blood bank. We had no time to warm it as we sent it scurrying down the IV tubing and into her jugular vein. What blood ran into her immediately ran out cold from her heart.

For whatever reason—the lighting, the suction, the inability of the sutures to take hold—we could not close the hole in her heart at the bedside. We needed to be in the OR, where we could operate in a more controlled environment. But a trip to the operating room meant maneuvering through two elevators and several long tortuous hallways. As you know, I have taken these "bed rides" before and they usually don't end well. As we navigated our way to the OR, my thighs, quivering with exhaustion, finally gave way owing to muscle fatigue. The anesthesiologist in tow had to literally hold me up by supporting my back so I could maintain my left hand position on Rosie's heart as we rode. I ignored the searing pain in my limbs that felt like branding irons, closed my eyes, and prayed all the way to the OR. I prayed quietly to myself, using the inner voice in my head, and then without knowing it, my lips began to move in silent prayer.

Every so often I would palpate her aorta to feel what her blood pressure was. It's a trick every cardiac surgeon knows. We develop, through touch alone, an uncanny ability to judge blood pressure. With one finger, I can gently touch the aorta and tell you within 3 to 5 mmHg what a patient's systolic blood pressure is. I could feel her aorta soften as her blood pressure sagged and I relayed this information to the anesthesiologist, who, with his one free hand, would increase the amount of epinephrine (adrenaline) we were pumping into her to maintain an adequate blood pressure. Despite all of the bleeding, Rosie's heart kept beating and never lost its rhythm. Such is the strength of the will to live.

When we made it to the operating room, everyone collectively exhaled. The OR, like a bunker in combat, provided us a safe haven as the bullets of Rosie's impending death sailed over our heads. We managed to get control of the bleeding and felt, for one brief glorious moment, a sense of victory. A gnawing, empty feeling in the pit of my stomach told me, however, that everything wasn't all right.

"Her pupils are fixed and dilated," the anesthesiologist pronounced. As if Rosie had heard this bit of lifeless information, her heart, within moments, ceased to beat and we could not restart it despite our best efforts.

"Can you close her up while I go talk to the family?" my surgical colleague said. He looked like a beaten man. "Sure. Of course," I sullenly replied. Someone had brought the cracking-the-chest cart to the operating room to restock it with OR supplies. And so I went to the cart. To that drawer. You know what drawer. That drawer. The unlabeled drawer. The bottom drawer. I removed three sternal wires from that vile drawer, which I would use to reapproximate the bone edges of her split sternum. I don't have to bring the bone together—I could just simply close the skin over the open bone—but I thought that it would look nicer if I brought the bone together. This is the least that I could do for Rosie. After her breastbone was closed, I then closed her skin in one swift layer using the No. 1 suture in an over-and-over whipstitch, or baseball stitch. The crudeness of this closure made it feel as though I were trussing a prime rib roast, not closing a young woman's chest.

It was a horrible feeling. A loathsome, sickening feeling and I longed to find some solace in the scene that lay before me. As I looked down upon Rosie, the first thing I noticed was her wedding ring, which only served to remind me that she was leaving behind not only a husband but a young son, Pierce. But then I saw it. Finally. A small source of comfort. Her hair. Her luxurious long blond hair that cascaded randomly over the white pillow beneath her head. Some strands had retained their golden yellow hue; others had been streaked with blood and matted together. Thin loose strands intermingled with thick clumped strands. It was her beauty. It was her chaos. It was Jackson Pollock.

13

The Bionic Woman

For christmas one year, when i was just a kid on the verge of becoming a teenager, my dad bought my mom a shiny new lawn mower. Not a particularly romantic gift, perhaps, but certainly very practical and very useful. He hid it in the garage on Christmas Eve and would surprise her with it in the morning. It was red and white—the colors of Christmas—and he adorned it with a simple silver bow. By our standards, it was a sophisticated machine. It had a self-propelling mechanism that made it easier to push than the old clunker of a mower that we shared with our grandfather next door. It even had a side bag attachment to catch the grass. "Yippeee!" my siblings and I thought. "No more raking." I remember thinking that I had never seen anything so beautiful. Perhaps it was the simple fact that it was new. Brand-new. Not the used, dented, scratched, secondhand, rebuilt machines that we were used to working with on the farm. Yes, to me, it was the Bentley of lawn mowers.

It was the eve of Christmas and I couldn't sleep. It wasn't, however, because of the anticipation of the coming morning but rather because someone was making an awful racket in the garage, which was directly below the bedroom I shared with my sister. Could it be Santa Claus? I tiptoed downstairs to the garage and slowly opened the door. And what to my wondering eyes should appear? My brother David, barely seven years old, taking apart my mother's new lawn mower. He had the entire mower completely disassembled and the parts were scattered on a green plaid blanket spread upon the garage floor. It looked like a picnic between two robots.

"What are you doing, David?" I exclaimed.

"I wanted to see how it worked," he said. His blue/brown eyes (he has one blue eye and one brown eye) looked up at me like an innocent doe's.

"You better put that thing back together or you're gonna get in big trouble," I warned and huffed back to bed.

By the morning, that lawn mower did not have so much as a fingerprint on it. There was not a single sign of the dissection that had gone on just hours before. This from my brother, a mechanical savant, who barely made it through high school even with the tireless kitchen table tutoring of my mother. He stuttered. He couldn't spell. Reading was a serious challenge. But this kid, this child, could take apart anything mechanical and put it back together with such intellect and alacrity that it bordered on genius.

Everyone in my family is mechanically inclined, although perhaps not to the level of David. This is in part due to genetics (my maternal grandfather was a handyman and my dad has an engineering degree) and necessity (our hand-me-down tractors and other machines were constantly in need of repair). I, too, have this love of all things mechanical, which explains why I get goose bumps at the sight of a "six-pack"— three two-barrel carburetors—hidden beneath the hood of a '66 GTO "goat." It also explains why I fell inexplicably in love with mechanical hearts, known as VADs—ventricular assist devices.

A VAD is an artificial heart much like dialysis is an artificial kidney. VADs are connected to the human heart and take over most, if not all, of its function. They are used in one of three ways: (1) They can allow the heart to rest after a massive injury such as a myocardial infarction, in hopes that the heart will eventually recover; (2) they can be used to bridge a patient who would otherwise die to a heart transplant while waiting on the transplant list for a suitable donor; and (3) they can be used as definitive therapy (known as destination therapy) in patients who do not qualify for a transplant. These patients live with their VAD indefinitely until they die of some other cause. Most of the VADs nowadays are fairly lightweight and not too cumbersome, so that patients can lead active lives. They just have to remember that, just like in a cell phone, they have to keep their batteries charged!

In 1998, the University of Pittsburgh Medical Center was one of the few transplant centers in the country that was offering formal training in VAD surgery during the year of heart/lung transplant fellowship. As a result, I became one of the few female VAD surgeons in the country. I was fascinated by these lifesaving machines and would spend hours with one of Pittsburgh's bioengineers, Steve, who was a brilliant and good-natured guy not unlike my brother, taking VADs apart to see how they ticked. They functioned with the simplicity of

the Tin Man's clock heart and yet had the design complexity
of a space station. I loved VADs as much as I loved a chromed-
out two-barrel carburetor.

Which is why, when I took my first real job (at the tender age of thirty-six!) after graduating from the Pittsburgh program, I took it upon myself to build a Mechanical Assist
Device program at my hospital using my recently acquired
knowledge and training. Aptly known as the MAD program, it
took just an ounce or so of insanity to begin a program of such
magnitude and complexity at the time I was just sharpening
my knives at my very first job. Especially when I hadn't really
established myself as a surgeon on staff yet. Talk about jumping in with both feet . . .

. . .

The first MAD call came after my third day on the job.

"Listen. I hear you're the new guy in cardiac surgery and
you can do these VAD things."

Silence on my end, then, "Yes . . ."

"Well, I got this lady here in the CCU. She's got familial
cardiomyopathy—the whole family's had it and died. She's
been in refractory VT and VF since she came in. We've
shocked her twenty-seven times so far this afternoon."

"What's she like now?"

"She's tubed, on drips, paralyzed with a balloon pump.
The whole nine yards."

"How are her organs holding up?"

"Well, her kidneys shut down. Last creatinine was 4.7
and she's not peeing. Liver numbers are sky-high in the thousands and her gases suck. She's not oxygenating. We've got her
on as much PEEP as her heart can handle at this point. She'll

probably blow a lung at any moment. Can't tell you how her squash is, though, since she's knocked out on Diprivan."

"Sounds like a train wreck."

"Yeah, a thirty-seven-year-old train wreck with three kids. Girls."

"I'll be right there. But just one more question. Where's the CCU?"

Click.

I was so brand-spanking new at the hospital that I didn't even know where the CCU—the coronary care unit—was and the *click* on the other end of the phone meant that I was on my own to find it. To make things even worse, the two most senior partners in the group of cardiothoracic surgeons I had just joined were out of town on vacation so I had no one with whom to really bounce off this consult. I guess I'd be truly finding my way all on my own. It was time for me to fly solo.

There is a crucial point in the life of a doctor when you must cut the umbilical cord between yourself and your mentors. The mentors who have protected you. Fed you. Kept you alive and perfused you with their knowledge and experience. Sometimes the transection is abrupt, as was the case with me. Other times there is a slow unraveling of the connection. In either case, though, it is like stepping out of a plane and not knowing for sure if your chute will open. I felt fear. I felt excitement. Then I felt more fear. But somehow I had to just lock it down . . . and . . . jump. During the free fall I reviewed all of my training, all of my hardships, all of my weaknesses and transgressions, my failures, my successes. I thought about my technical skill set, my intellect, my ability to make good judgments and quick descisions, my God-given ability to heal.

I thought about the people who had supported me along the way. The ones, especially my family, who had unwavering confidence in me. And that is when my chute opened and I drifted confidently above the scene at hand knowing that I could, if given the chance, independently save a life. Because to finally be an autonomously functioning attending surgeon, this severance must take place. Otherwise you will always be what surgeons call a "boy." A boy is a surgeon who isn't good enough to operate on her own and must stay in the shadow of an older, more experienced surgeon. If this happens, it will kill any hope you had of gaining the respect of the cardiologists who might have referred cases to you, because eventually they see you only as a shadow—a dark silhouette of a surgeon without form, function, or substance. That's why a surgeon must take the plunge.

I arrived at the patient's bedside and stood at the foot of her bed, the best vantage point from which to survey the situation. My hands gripped the foot of the bed as I took in the view before me. A gale force wind could not have pried me loose. She was exactly as billed.

Lying supine upon the bed, connected to a ventilator, Lindsey was loosely covered only in a blue and white patterned hospital gown to her knees. She lay motionless save for the regular rise and fall of her chest as the ventilator blew oxygen-rich air into and out of her lungs. The lines etched on her face in a deep pattern around her eyes and mouth made her look older than her stated age. She had lived the hard life of familial cardiomyopathy—a hereditary cardiac disorder that causes profound heart failure at a young age, when most people feel invincible and take life for granted.

Congestive heart failure (CHF), or the inability of the heart to pump blood effectively, affects five million people in the United States and twenty-three million people worldwide; as such, it is the most common admitting diagnosis for any patient at any hospital in the United States. It is responsible for more than one million hospital admissions per year. Once diagnosed with CHF, 70 percent of women under the age of sixty-five will die within eight years. When a patient progresses to class IV, or late-stage heart failure, his or her life expectancy is just one year. Lindsey was in late-stage heart failure and her life hung in the balance. So, too, do the lives of the nearly thirty-two thousand women who die annually of CHF. This lone vicious killer is responsible for 62.6 percent of all heart disease–related deaths in women.

Lindsey's CCU room, although normally quite sweeping, seemed small because of the clutter of life support equipment—seven IVAC infusion pumps that delivered a constant stream of intravenous cardiac medications called inotropes; a dialysis machine already taking over for her now-defunct kidneys; the balloon pump that inflated and deflated inside her aorta, which served as a temporary measure to help her heart propel blood forward and also perfuse her coronary arteries; and the ever-present ventilator cranking out PEEP—positive end expiratory pressure—to inflate her lungs. The room was dimly lit so as to give the false impression of calm and serenity because the smallest amount of stimulation would cause an adrenaline rush in Lindsey and flip her heart into the lethal VT/VF (ventricular tachycardia/ventricular fibrillation) rhythm. To me, however, the blinking lights and sounds of all of the equipment made it look like a macabre carnival of sorts.

"We're gonna need an OR and a miracle," was all I said to the cardiologist who stood, Red Bull in hand, intently watching me survey the room.

As it turned out, I was wrong. I needed more than an OR

and a miracle. Much more. I needed a VAD. The hospital didn't have two of the types of VAD that I was accustomed to using at Pittsburgh, so we needed to procure one off the shelves of a nearby university hospital. Since VADs cost somewhere north of sixty-four thousand dollars, this was no easy feat, but you can't put a price tag on life (unless, of course, you are a health insurance company).

Equipment in hand, we headed off to the OR to implant not one but two "carburetors" into the heart's chassis, because both the left and right sides of Lindsey's heart had failed and both sides needed assistance with a VAD. The surgery was a success (big sigh of relief here) and we rolled out of the OR twelve hours later with a much more stable patient.

Remember, this was my first solo flight as an attending surgeon. It was the first time I had implanted a VAD without having an experienced surgeon talking me through the operation. In fact, the surgeon I was operating with hadn't really seen this type of implant procedure. Thankfully, before I left Pittsburgh, I had written down, in sequence, the hundreds of steps needed to implant a VAD. I kept this information in a notebook, which I had quickly reviewed, in the sanctity of the ladies' bathroom outside the OR, before the surgery. Each step had to be performed in a precise, well-thought-out order since, like building a house of cards, each move was dependent on the move preceding it.

After the surgery, I was so worried about Lindsey that I slept in the ICU in a room next to hers and stayed by her side all night. The VAD was cranking out five to six liters per minute of nourishing blood flow to her starving organs throughout the night. By the following morning, Lindsey was awake and was being weaned from the ventilator. The day after that, her kidney function had recovered to the point of no longer needing dialysis and her liver function was normalizing. It was the miracle I needed. The miracle I had prayed for.

On the third morning after surgery, I wanted to get Lindsey out of bed and I instructed the nurses to do this with the help of two superb physical therapists, Leslie and Cassie. I returned to Lindsey's room later that afternoon only to be told that the patient hadn't gotten out of bed.

"Why didn't you get her up?" I asked the nurses taking care of Lindsey.

No one answered me. They just stared at their feet and wouldn't make eye contact with me. Finally, one nurse whispered, "We thought they'd fall out."

"What would fall out?" I replied.

"The VADs," she replied.

The act of implanting an artificial heart requires that you marry man (or, in this case, woman) to a machine. This union has to be perfect because in this relationship one cannot function properly without the other. As such, there are two competing elements to the operation—the human element and the mechanical element. The human heart has to be prepared to accept the machine and the machine has to be assembled in such a way as to be accepted by the heart.

During surgery, the human body is much more gracious and forgiving than is the VAD. The human body is extremely complex, with redundancy built in so that it can compensate, to a certain extent, for inaccuracies in surgical technique—much like a blind person who acquires a heightened sense of smell, sound, and taste to better cope. The VAD, however, is a very simple machine—whatever volume of blood is drawn into the machine is pumped out, matching input to output. It is not very good at compensating for inadequate flow in either direction and so precision at implant is crucial. One small misstep, one missed detail, the slightest kink or torsion makes all the difference between a successful and an unsuccessful implant.

I had inserted two VADs, known as a BiVAD, which were extracorporeal, into Lindsey. This meant that each VAD was connected to the heart in two places by long tubes, or cannulas. The cannulas are then tunneled under the skin of the upper abdomen, where they exit the skin and are connected to the actual pumping chamber of the VAD, which sits outside the body (extracorporeal) and lies flat against the patient's abdomen. To the untrained eye, it looks as though there is nothing holding the VAD in place. It appears to just dangle from the skin. This is why the nurses thought it would fall out when the patient stood up.

"But haven't you seen a BiVAD patient before?" I asked the nurses.

"Yes. Only a few. But we've never seen one live long enough to get out of bed."

And just like that—with one success—my MAD program was born.

The nurses were so amazed and excited to see Lindsey recover that they actually fought over who would get to take care of her and get her out of bed. Once we were past this hurdle of merely getting Lindsey out of bed, we quickly worked toward having her walk on her own. Watching this dying, bedridden woman take her first steps was no less moving than seeing your own toddler take his. As we became more confident in the technology, we became a more adventurous group. We took Lindsey on walks all around the hospital. The VAD ran on batteries while we moved about and when we stopped to rest, we would plug Lindsey into a wall socket. (One nurse's job, Bernard, was to carry a long extension cord just in case!) We even ventured outdoors so that Lindsey could feel the healing California sun on her face and fill her recovering lungs with warm Pacific air.

With each step that Lindsey took, she grew stronger and my MAD program grew stronger. We came together as a team—nurses, doctors, physical therapists, nutritionists, respiratory therapists. A MAD team. And boy, did we save lives! One after the other we pulled patients back from the brink of death with our VADs to live to see another day. And another. And another. Like Lindsey, they would successfully bridge to a heart transplant and watch their children grow up. The nurses had a name for it—AKM, which stood for Another Kathy Miracle. But it wasn't my miracle, it was *our* miracle. Our MAD miracle. And to think it all began with one solo flight. One bionic woman. One ounce of courage and equal parts insanity. I am proud to say that the Mechanical Assist Device program at that hospital is alive and well today.

So, too, is Lindsey.

14

Torn Apart

We are waiting. We are standing in the ambulance bay outside the ED—the Emergency Department—and we are waiting. Incidentally, it offends every emergency care physician to call it an ER because, as they will gladly correct you, "We are a department, *not* a room." Please be respectful of this the next time you set foot in an ER . . . ED. And yes, I, too, have made this faux pas in all the preceding chapters.

We are waiting. Waiting for sirens. Waiting for lights. Waiting for the challenge that will inevitably emerge from the ambulance unbidden. We are giddy with anticipation, like children waiting for the best ride in the amusement park, my surgical comrades and I, for incoming was a forty-nine-year-old with an aortic dissection. We pace. We check our Black-Berrys, we pace some more.

In my head I am doing the math. *Okay. If she arrives here in the next five minutes, it will be fifteen thirty-five hours. (Surgeons always use military time. I guess it's because we always feel as though we are in battle.) Get her out of the ambulance; wheel her to ICU for a blood draw and a consent form. Can take the history and physical on the way to the unit. If the OR's ready for us—big "if" here—we're in there by sixteen hundred hours, give or take. Now factor in the anesthesia prep time for lines and tubes, then we're asleep by seventeen hundred hours and ready to cut skin by seventeen fifteen. If the procedure goes without a hitch, then we're out by . . .*

I'm doing this calculation in my head to see if there is any way in hell I'll see my kids tonight. "Not a chance" is the result of my summation. So I call my son Nicholas to tell him that Mommy won't be home tonight.

"How come?" he asks.

"Because I have an aortic dissection," I answer, hoping to satisfy his curiosity.

It never works. He's too bright a kid.

"What's that?" he asks.

"Well, honey, it's where the heart explodes a little."

"Does blood come shooting out?"

"No, honey, it really sort of just tears."

There is a pause and I can tell he is turning this new information over in his mind, trying to find a grasp.

"Like when your sock tears and your toe pokes out?"

"Yes," I lie, "exactly like that."

After all, one must protect the frailty of a five-year-old.

• • •

Although her face was weathered by time, her eyes were filled with the brightness of youth. You could just tell that she was a woman who was used to being in control of her life and even her destiny. I knew that the conversation I was about to have with her would be the most difficult of her life. It would test her limits.

Her name was Esther and she was ninety-four years old (not forty-nine, as some dyslexic dispatcher had told us), having just celebrated her birthday a few months earlier, in August. Although she had no children, her friends and neighbors called her Grandma. When I introduced myself to her in the Emergency Department, she took my hand, looked me in the eye with her bright gaze, and said, "Call me Grandma, dear, and tell me how I am going to die."

She had presented at the ED with twenty-four hours of steady chest pressure that began in her midchest behind her breastbone. The pain, dull at first, grew steadier and sharper until it felt like a "tearing" sensation that radiated to her back and between her shoulder blades. She ignored the pain at first but, as the day progressed and the pain overcame her, she knew that it meant something ominous was happening. She knew it meant her unavoidable death. And so she ignored it, content to die alone at home surrounded by her things and mementos of her life. It wasn't until her best friend and neighbor, Chavez, stopped by and insisted that she go to the hospital that she reluctantly made her way into my care. To die. By the time she was finally admitted to the Emergency Department, her blood pressure was dangerously low. Her kidneys had failed and were making no urine. Her liver was shutting down. Her extremities were cold, clammy, and pulseless.

We obtained a CAT scan and an echocardiogram, both of which confirmed her diagnosis. She had an ascending aortic dissection, and without emergency surgery she was going to die. Today. Within a few hours.

An aortic dissection is a tear in the lining of the greatest blood vessel that leaves the heart, the aorta. The aorta carries all of the oxygen-rich blood, which is pumped from the left side of the heart, to all parts of the body. An aortic dissection is like a run in a stocking. All it takes is one small tear to start an uncontrollable process that essentially rips the layers of the aorta apart lengthwise, proximally to distally. This process "shears off" all of the tributary arteries that send blood from the aorta to the organs and extremities. The organs die of blood deprivation, taking the patient with them.

Esther needed emergency surgery to repair the tear and restore blood flow. The surgery was extremely high risk, with a small hope of survival given her age and her state of organ failure. But without surgery, there was *no* hope of survival. It was her choice.

When I approached her gurney to get her final decision, she was surrounded by her friends, who were all pleading with her to have the operation. All except Chavez. He was the only one who smiled at me as I approached. He was calm. He was the only one besides the patient who didn't look distraught. I knelt down beside her so that she and I could see eye to eye. I asked her if she wanted to undergo surgery. She fully understood the risks and benefits of the procedure. She understood the consequences of not having surgery.

Of course, I knew her answer. "No, thank you," is what she said, with those youthful eyes locked on mine. She said it as if I had just offered her a cup of tea. I've learned that accepting one's own death can be a very comfortable and natural decision for some people. For others, it is a decision filled with struggle and anger to be wrestled with using all of their might. For Esther, it was almost cathartic. I could see the relief in her eyes. I will never forget those eyes.

We admitted her to a private hospital room. The hospice team attended to making her comfortable. I went back to my office but couldn't shake the thought of her. A few hours later,

I received a call from the hospice nurses saying that Esther was "almost gone." I dropped what I was doing and ran to her bedside. I was surprised to find her alone. She had sent her friend Chavez, who had been a constant fixture at her side, to her house to bring back a few things from her home to brighten her room. Her favorite ceramic vases. Her colorful African tribal masks.

When I entered her room, I knew Death was imminent because I could smell it. Death has a distinct odor. It smells like wet metal. I can only describe it as the smell you would encounter if just after a rainfall you were walking past the steel girders of a building being erected. It is a stale odor that is not pungent but rather lingers faintly in the background of other aromas contained in a room. It is hardly perceptible. I suppose this is because Death often likes to arrive unnoticed. Unheralded. Like a guest who is unfashionably early for a party, Death likes to slip in among the other visitors before anyone has a chance to notice he is present. Seldom is he invited, he simply assumes that, eventually, everyone will want him there. Such is his prowess. When the other guests see Death—guests like Pain, who is doubled over in the corner; Grief, the puddle in the middle of the room; and Sadness, hiding pathetically within the shadow of the door—they all look away for fear that they might make eye contact with him. Although Death shows up without an escort, he never leaves the party alone.

He always takes Life with him, clinging to his arm, when he departs.

And so there I was, sitting beside this dying woman as she lay peacefully in bed. Her breathing was very shallow now. I had to look closely at her chest to see if indeed she was still breathing. She was very comfortable. No more tearing. No more pain. Her head, gently turned to the left, was pressed into the three soft pillows that were beneath her. Her arms were relaxed at her sides, palms down, fingers gently resting on the white bed linens. At her bedside table was a half-filled glass of Coca-Cola and the empty can. A small triangle of dark chocolate—the corner broken off a candy bar—was next to the soda. I could see that she had nibbled the edge. When I saw the chocolate, I smiled, thinking that her last taste of life was bittersweet. Appropriately so.

I sat on the bed next to her. A position I have assumed a thousand times before when talking with patients. But there was no discussion. Just silent prayer. I watched her breathe until her breath was no more. As death overtook her, her body relaxed more, making a deeper indentation into the pillows, the mattress.

Just then, Chavez entered the room. "You just couldn't wait for me, could you?" he said to Esther. His arms were laden with vases and masks. He and I stayed in her room together for quite some time. We sat in silence and I comforted him as best I could. It was a time for closure. A time to spend with what was physically left behind, her body, and say good-bye because her spirit had already left the room. When I finally decided to leave her room, Chavez gave me one of her bright orange vases, which I have in my home. As with all the other women with cardiovascular disease whom I have treated and who have died, I think of her often.

· · ·

An aortic dissection is an old enemy. King George II of England, Lucille Ball, and more recently John Ritter all died from them.

It occurs in two out of every ten thousand people and is found in 1 to 2.5 percent of all autopsies. One-third of patients die within the first twenty-four hours and half die within forty-eight hours. Aortic dissections are caused by a tear in the inner lining of the aorta known as the intimal layer. This causes blood to extravasate, or leak out, between the layers within the wall of the aorta, which causes a false lumen to propagate, like having a tube within a tube. The inner lumen is the true lumen and the outer lumen is a false channel. This false lumen reduces and even eliminates blood flow to all the major tributary arteries that branch off the aorta. The tear can also cause a free rupture of the aorta, which, when it occurs, causes patients to bleed to death within seconds.

Like most enemies, aortic dissections come in many forms. They are classified medically by where the origin of the tear occurs in the aorta. The classification is known as the Stanford classification. If the tear occurs in the ascending or beginning of the aorta, it is classified as a Type A dissection. If the tear occurs at a point beyond the ascending aorta, it is called a Type B dissection. This classification is important because it guides our treatment decision.

Aortic dissections have no valor. No pride. They like to prey upon the weak and the frail. Any woman is at risk for a dissection when the wall of her aorta naturally weakens and degenerates with age and with atherosclerosis. Certain diseases such as Marfan syndrome, Ehlers-Danlos syndrome, and polycystic kidney disease can predispose women to aortic dissection. Women with high blood pressure are especially at risk as well as women with an abnormal aortic valve known as a bicuspid aortic valve. Aortic dissection can be precipitated by pregnancy, syphilis, cocaine use, or a severe blow to the chest, such as hitting the steering wheel during a motor vehicle accident. Half of all dissections in women under the age of forty are due to pregnancy. The peak age for a dissection is fifty to sixty-nine years old and it is seen more commonly in African Americans.

Aortic dissections are a swift enemy but are essentially cowards at heart because they like to hide themselves from physicians and are often misdiagnosed. The most common symptom of an aortic dissection is pain that usually begins in the chest. The pain is very sudden in onset, often waking a patient from sleep. It is described as "ripping or tearing" pain, which usually migrates to the patient's back. A person undergoing an aortic dissection will often say that he "felt like someone was stabbing him in the back." The pain is usually maximal at onset, unlike that of a heart attack, which usually builds up gradually. The source of the pain will often change as the dissection rips the aorta distally. For example, the pain may move from the chest and back to the neck and jaw and then to the lower back and flank.

As the tributary arteries lose their blood flow, symptoms other than pain arise. Symptoms of a stroke can emerge, such as altered mental status and limb weakness, pain, or paralysis. Five percent of patients will have a fainting episode. Hoarseness and difficulty swallowing are also seen. Patients often become profoundly short of breath and cannot lie flat. They are often extremely anxious and, oddly, will describe a feeling of "doom" or a premonition of death.

The key to fighting this enemy is to find it first. One of its best defense mechanisms is mimicry, which it uses to deceive physicians trying to make a diagnosis. Unfortunately, aortic dissections are sly and are often mistaken for other diseases. Blood studies and an EKG are performed to rule out a heart attack, which often can mimic an aortic dissection in its presentation. A chest X-ray is the quickest and easiest imaging study and will show some abnormality related to a dissection 80 percent of the time. However, there are four other imaging studies that we have in our armamentarium to definitively diagnose an aortic dissection: an angiogram, an echocardiogram, a computer-assisted tomography (CAT) scan, and a magnetic resonance imaging (MRI) scan.

There are two strategies we can use to defeat an aortic dissection before it kills. One is a medical tactic and the other is a surgical tactic. The immediate medical treatment for an aortic dissection is to control the blood pressure and heart rate to try to stop the tear from progressing and causing the aorta to freely rupture. The goal is to keep the systolic blood pressure, or higher blood pressure number, between 90 and 110 mmHg and the heart rate between sixty and seventy beats per minute. This is done with intravenous medication. If the imaging tests reveal that a patient has a Type B aortic dissection, then this type of medical care is all the patient needs unless her blood pressure and heart rate cannot be controlled or the dissection worsens and progresses.

A surgical tactic is used for a Type A dissection. The surgical treatment for aortic dissections is one of the most challenging emergency operations that I perform. The goal of surgery is to find the tear and fix it by replacing the torn segment of the aorta with a segment of synthetic graft material. Although this seems like a simple endeavor, in reality it is not. The tear often causes injury to the aortic valve, coronary arteries, and great vessels which supply blood to the brain. All of these will also need to be repaired and/or replaced, which complicates the procedure. The procedure is often done under "total circulatory arrest." During total circulatory arrest, the patient's body is cooled to approximately 18 degrees C (64 degrees F) by the heart-lung machine. The patient's head and open chest are packed in ice for additional cooling. This profoundly cold state is incompatible with life and puts the patients into a kind of hibernation. The cold temperature lowers the body's metabolism to a near lifeless state. All of the patient's blood is drained into the heart-lung machine and the machine is then turned off. For all intents and purposes, the patient is clinically dead. No heartbeat, no respiration. Her brain waves, monitored by EEG, are flatline and the patient has no blood in her body. This allows us to work in a bloodless field to repair the aorta. The patient can be in this suspended animation state for approximately forty to fifty minutes; if it takes any longer, she is less likely to "come back." When the operation is complete, the blood is returned to the patient's body and she is slowly warmed to a normal temperature. When the body reaches a normal temperature, the heart, with its will to live, begins to beat and the patient's organs all begin to function. The patient is then weaned from the heart-lung machine.

I am in awe of circulatory arrest. If there is a *Twilight Zone* in medicine, this is certainly it. Whenever we turn off the heart-lung machine, and open the aorta without seeing the inevitable torrent of blood that should gush forth, I always take a look over my shoulder to see if Rod Serling is standing behind me. And where do these people, drained of their blood, go when they are under circulatory arrest without brain, heart, or lung function? Do they hover above us like observers in an OR amphitheater, peering into their own gaping chest cavities? Do they visit with loved ones who have passed away while teetering on the fine line between life and death? Are they sitting in a lounge chair on a cloud with their feet up, martini in hand, watching a documentary of their life as it passes before them? I like to imagine that they are in Iowa, wandering through the fields of wheat with hands outstretched at their sides, allowing their fingertips to be tickled by the tips of the golden shafts. Why Iowa and wheat fields? Because it's something solid and concrete that I can focus on in the middle of an operation and because that's just the kind of quirky setting that Rod Serling would have portrayed.

• • •

When I finally arrived home that day (or the next, really) in the cool darkness of 0300, having suffered through the last moments of Esther's long, fulfilling life, there was a drawing left for me by Nicholas on the kitchen table. It was a picture of a heart with a jagged crack in it centered on a sheet of white paper. There were many arcing lines speading outward from the heart to the edges of the paper. At the end of each line was either another smaller heart with no crack in it or else the words "I love you, Mommy." In the morning, a mere three hours later, Nicholas explained the drawing to me.

"It's an aortic dissection," he says confidently. I was impressed that he remembered the name of the disease. He explained further that when the heart explodes, "love" (the "I love yous") and "joy" (the smaller healed hearts) come out.

"Because when you really, really love me, Mommy," he explains, "you say that your heart is bursting with love and joy for me."

"Yes," I say, without a single shred of a lie this time. "I do."

15

The Seat of the Soul

I AM RELANDSCAPING MY FRONT YARD. AGAIN. FOR THE third time. It's very frustrating. Every time I plant anything green in that yard it dies. I cannot keep green things alive. If a Martian were to fall from the sky and land upon the earth, he would die at my feet. Why? Because he's green.

Thank God my patients are all pink or, well, gray really. Gray because they are not pumping enough blood to their skin. Even though your skin is technically the largest organ in (or on) your body, it's not a priority for blood supply. Brain, heart, and kidneys take precedence. That is why, when you're dying on my operating table, you're gray. And thank God for that because *you* I can save. If you were even the slightest shade of green during the throes of death, you'd be a goner in my book.

Last week my husband and I were with our landscape designer, Jill, selecting plants from an abundant nursery in Vista. We've decided to plant all succulents and cacti to be more environmentally friendly. That, and maybe these guys will have a chance at survival. Kelly, the gentleman who oversees the nursery, drove us around in a golf cart as we oohed and aahed over the plants. They were amazing specimens— each unique in its presentation. Whenever he drove past a plant he particularly liked, he would stop, get out of the cart, and kneel down next to it. He would gently and cautiously caress the plant (especially if it was a spiny cactus) and tell us the plant's origin, genus, and species. Where its native country was and how he'd grown it from a seed or sapling. He did this so many times that it suddenly dawned on me that the whole place, acres and acres, was his. It was his life's work— growing all these plants from seeds. Nurturing them. Caring for them. Protecting them. Each and every plant.

How amazing, I thought, to be able to walk among the totality of your life's work. To see it all laid out before you and survey its glory. I wish I could have that. A garden filled with all of the patients whom I have devoted my life to. All of the lives that I have touched in some way. Those whom I have nurtured and cared for. Those whom I have saved.

To think that I could walk among them all and tell you their origin, genus, species or, rather, their illness, their operation, their recovery. To walk among my life's work. To take a moment to stop at each one and touch her or him gently. My hands cupping each face or resting on a shoulder. My palm pressing oh so delicately against an incision. To connect with them in some way and tell them all that I am truly honored to have been a part of their lives and the lives of their families and friends.

That would be a great moment.

A moment like that happened to me just recently, albeit

on a much smaller scale. Though this story is about a male patient of mine, it could just as easily be about any woman facing a heart transplant.

I was out at dinner with some friends of mine from the hospital. It was my birthday and they said they had a surprise for me. Just as we were seated, in walked Sylvester with his wife, Jackie. Seeing him walking tall and steady toward me, not wearing a soiled hospital gown, not having a feeding tube protruding snakelike from his stomach or an endotracheal tube hanging from his cracked and bleeding lips, his skin not hideously bruised with small black and blue disks that coalesced from the hundreds of needlesticks he endured, walking upright, not lying in bed for weeks on end while the muscles of his lower extremities atrophied until all that was left of his legs was skin and bones, not coding, not dying, gave me great pause and took me back to my birthday six years before, when I had given Sylvester his heart. He and his wife are two of the most amazing flowers in my healing garden. To dine with the two of them, and revel in how healthy Sylvester was, was a great birthday gift and indeed a great moment.

He gently took my hand and we sat down to a simple dinner—an act that would have been unimaginable six years earlier. During the nine months that I took care of him, Sylvester had six separate cardiac and respiratory arrests. I first met him in December, when while in California to escape the cold of the East Coast and be at the birth of his first grandchild, he developed angina. Sylvester was sixty-three years old and was the president and founder of a company that manufactured acoustic products for offices. He was thinking about semiretiring and spending more time with his devoted wife of forty-four years, slowing down and taking time to enjoy life. The fact that he had angina was no surprise to him. He had had bypass surgery in the 1970s and stents (tiny metal tubes that are placed inside a coronary artery to hold the artery open) inserted in the 1990s. Yes, he was no stranger to cardiovascular disease. It's just that, like most people, he thought he would live forever even with heart disease. And besides, he had no time to be ill. He had a grandchild on the way and there was much to do.

When the pain, which he described as a boring pain and pressure deep in the center of his chest, "as if an elephant were sitting on me," became unrelenting, he finally came into the hospital. A cardiac catheterization confirmed that he needed repeat bypass surgery and one of my partners was asked to do it. Some of his vessels were less than one millimeter in diameter and therefore could not be bypassed. For those territories within the heart in which a new bypass graft could not be introduced, the cardiac surgeon would perform TMR. Transmyocardial revascularization is a technique in which we drill tiny holes in the muscle of the heart with a laser to allow blood to penetrate these areas.

At the conclusion of the case, the surgeon seemed quite pleased with how Sylvester was doing. Within thirty-six hours of the operation, however, he was in full cardiac arrest. He was brought back to the OR and I was called in to assess the situation. As I peered into his open chest, I could clearly see that the heart was struggling. Large swaths of muscle were injured. The muscle was beefy red and edematous and not contracting. He was in cardiogenic shock and his heart was not strong enough to save him. In fact, his heart was killing him.

Sylvester needed to have two mechanical hearts implanted to stabilize him. Without these, he would never be weaned from the heart-lung machine and would die on the table. A heart transplant was in his future because this was not a heart that would ever recover. The BiVAD implant was a long and difficult surgery. On two occasions I had had to leave the OR to tell his family that I didn't think he would make it out of the operating room alive and they needed to prepare themselves. We held hands there in the waiting room and their strength flowed through me. We grasped one another's hands tightly the way you would if someone were dangling from a tenth-floor balcony. Not wanting to let go. Not wanting him to slip away and plummet to his death. Tightly. With desperation and fear. We held hands; white knuckled and in silence, we hoped. We prayed. As I turned to leave and make my way back to the OR, Jackie slipped a picture of their new granddaughter into my scrub shirt pocket and said, "Tell him he needs to live for her."

Barney Clark was the first person ever to receive a successful artificial/mechanical heart implant, the Jarvik-7 heart. It was 1982, exactly fifteen years after the first successful human heart transplant. Barney, a mild-mannered dentist from Des Moines, lay dying in his hospital bed with his wife ever present at his side. When the surgical team discussed the experimental surgery with his wife—that they would be removing his heart and replacing it with a machine—she asked but one question of the team:

"If you take out my husband's heart, will he still be able to love me?"

Such is the strength of the association between love and the human heart. Her only worry, after being told a laundry list of possible complications from this as yet untried procedure, was that if a machine replaced her husband's heart then perhaps his ability to love, not his will to love, would somehow be lost in the process. Many of my transplant patients take this one step further and ask:

"If you take my heart from my chest and in its place put another, will I lose my soul?"

When I replace a patient's heart with a donor heart, is the recipient taking the new soul of the deceased donor? Does it then become the recipient's job to house this soul? To feed it, nurture it, give it a new perch within her chest? Every morning a heart transplant patient greets the day looking at the scar upon her chest and wondering about the soul she has taken in and given sanctuary. Such is the joy, the fear, and the blessing that comes with being a heart transplant patient because the heart, a universal symbol of love, is also considered by many to be the seat of the soul.

Sylvester survived the implant of two VADs and began the slow, day-to-day, moment-to-moment journey down the road to a heart transplant. A journey often fraught with hills and valleys; twists and turns; treacherous passages; and long, dark tunnels waiting for the day when his new heart and soul would come. Each day was a challenge and he endured many complications while waiting nearly two months for an organ. Every time the helicopter lifted off from the heliport, he would ask, "Is it my turn? Is it going out for me?"

According to the UNOS (United Network of Organ Sharing) website as of July 31, 2009, there are 2,869 people waiting for a heart transplant. The number of people waiting for a kidney is 80,384; liver, 15,892; pancreas, 1,505; lung, 1,902; both a heart and lung, 84; and intestine, 228.

Just waiting. Just dying.

Sylvester's organ came from a college student in his early twenties who accidentally fell from a great height. He fell to the earth and crushed his skull, causing his brain to die, while the remainder of his body was miraculously spared. This one brain-dead donor saved or improved the lives of eleven perfect strangers:

1. *The corneas from his eyes would go to a fourteen-year-old blind girl robbed of her sight by a corneal perforation. She would see her parents again.*

2. *His skin would be used to temporarily graft a fireman who had third-degree burns over 60 percent of his body sustained during the rescue of a family of four from their burning home.*

3. *His bones, tendons, cartilage, and ligaments would be used as grafts to salvage the legs of a boy his age who sustained severe injuries during a car accident so that he might walk again.*

4. *& 5. His lungs, each one, would go to twin boys who are dying together from pulmonary fibrosis.*

6. *His pancreas and one kidney would save a thirty-eight-year-old lifelong brittle diabetic whose dream of going to graduate school would at last be realized.*

7. *His other kidney would save a mother of two from dialysis three times per week so she could go back to raising her children.*

8. *& 9. His liver would be split in two with the smaller left lateral segment going to a baby born with biliary atresia*

and not likely to see her first birthday. The larger right segment would go to a high school English teacher with hepatitis C.

10. His small intestine would be given to a child with an abnormally short bowel who is dying from malnutrition.

11. His heart, wrapped in the protective covering of the soul, would save Sylvester.

One donor can change—no, make that *save*—the world. What if the recipient of that lung goes on to find the cure for cancer? What if the recipient of that kidney goes on to develop an alternative clean energy source that can power all forms of transportation? What if the liver recipient achieves world peace? One donor can change the world, one recipient at a time.

If you are a donor, have known anyone who has donated an organ or, at the very least, has a signed donor card, then I must say two words to you: Thank you.

Thank you. Thank you. Thank you.

These two little words were what I was thinking as I landed at the heliport on the roof of the hospital with Sylvester's new heart safely stowed, packed in ice in a red Coleman beer cooler. As I rounded the corner to the OR, I ran smack into Jackie. She looked at me, then the cooler. I gave her a wink and a thumbs-up. She mouthed the words back to me that I was just thinking: "Thank you."

When the clock struck midnight fours hours later, the OR sang "Happy Birthday" to me. We started the transplant on March 3 but finished on March 4. My birthday. I was thirty-nine years old. Best damn birthday I ever had, except the one I had as a kid when my mom and dad got me a little green turtle.

I can always tell when a heart likes its new environment, that the souls, if you will, are compatible. Before I can get the last stitches in, the donor heart will start to beat spontaneously with no coaxing from me. It beats with the rhythm of a heart that has found its rebirth in its new home. This was exactly the case with Sylvester's heart—it leapt in his chest.

Sylvester spent the next seven months in the hospital recovering. His postoperative course was rocky at best. He had respiratory failure and required a tracheostomy. He had nutritional depletion and needed to have a feeding tube inserted directly into his stomach. He had blood sugar issues and kidney problems. One of his vocal cords became paralyzed and he had to learn to speak again. He arrested several times from various causes, one of which was a pulmonary embolism. When he was placed on powerful immunosuppressant medications, he convulsed in bed like something in a scene from a William Friedkin movie. All of this he endured with his beloved Jackie always at his bedside. Always under her watchful and loving eye. For better, for worse. In sickness and in health.

When he was finally discharged from the hospital after nine months, it was like I had given birth to a baby. A new life that I would send out into the world to make a difference. And here that new life sat next to me, in this restaurant, on my birthday, grazing on a salad. It blew my mind. It made *my* heart leap in *my* chest.

And so I asked Sylvester, "What do you remember about those nine months?"

"It was mostly a blur," he replied. "Maybe it was just because of all the medicine I was taking, but most of it now seems so unclear and far away.

"I do remember one very clear detail, though. I remember a light and a great blackness all around. And a hand . . . a woman's hand . . . pulling me back."

16

Where Have All the Good Times Gone?

It is not the strongest of the species that survive, or the most intelligent, but the one most responsive to change.

—Charles Darwin

W E DON'T CALL THEM VIPs ANYMORE. NOW THEY ARE referred to as PONs—persons of note. My first PON patient was a Hollywood mogul. A legend. Master of the studio executive universe. I was excited to meet him not because he was a PON but because I heard that he had fired one of the most prominent cardiologists at my hospital. I thought that was great. It took balls. The other stuff about him was icing on the cake because when you go under my knife, you are all equal. Who you are, what you do for a living, how much money you make, and how many important people you know are immaterial to me. I treat all patients like they are my family and my family members are all PONs.

After he fired his cardiologist, he began demanding to see "the surgeon." Well, I was busy and couldn't get up to his room to see him until late in the afternoon. As he waited, his anger grew and by the time I got to the floor, the nurses were all rolling their eyes at me. I walked briskly into his room, loaded for bear. I sat down on his bed beside him, immediately invading his space, and delivered my line. "So I hear you're pissed," I said, without so much as blinking. "Who the fuck are you?" was his response, holding my gaze. I loved him already. He had me at "fuck." "I'm the heart surgeon you've been waiting for all afternoon," I said, and then paused, waiting for what I thought would be the inevitable response from him. I expected the librarian-type comment or some other clever statement that basically says, "There must be some mistake. You're a woman and can't possibly be my surgeon. Please get a male surgeon, preferably with gray hair and a higher-than-thou attitude." It never came. He accepted me for who I was. Instantly. No questions asked. Later on, he told me it was because the "I hear you're pissed" line was such a great opener that he just couldn't resist having me operate on him. I'd like to think, however, it was because he likened me to Meg Ryan à la *City of Angels*. I get that association a lot from patients who meet me. And, yes, I wish I were as cute as she is.

Dan was a tough nut to crack. Literally. Opening his chest took hours and hours of tedious work because he had had pericarditis (an inflammation of the sac around the heart) years ago, which left the inside of his chest filled with scar tissue. When Michelangelo sculpted, he believed that he could see the image of a sculpture embedded in a block of marble and he would simply just remove the excess around it to achieve his artwork. This was what Dan's thoracic cavity was like. I knew there was a heart in there somewhere—a great big beautiful heart—but I had to spend hours chipping away at it to find any identifiable structures. The surgery ultimately took eleven hours, and I performed six

bypass grafts and a "maze" procedure to treat a chronic underlying erratic heartbeat. He often asks me why I didn't do
seven bypass grafts, to which I smile and answer, "I was too
tired to throw another one in."

The hospital billed Dan's insurance company for the cost
of his hospital stay and a separate procedure code, known as a
CPT code, was used for my surgical work. CPT, or current pro-
cedural terminology, codes were established by the American
Medical Association. They describe medical, surgical, or diagnostic services, which communicate uniform information
among doctors, hospitals, billing personnel, and most important, insurance companies. It's a numeric language of sorts.
An ingrown toenail, or onychocryptosis, as it is known in po-
diatric medicine, has a CPT code of 11730, which stands for
"removal of nail plate." When your foot doctor removes your
ingrown nail, he submits code 11730 to your insurance company. Attached to that individual code is a dollar amount that
the insurance company will pay the doctor (for this code, the
payment is $52.38). But the insurance company will *not* pay
the doctor unless an ICD-9 code is also submitted with the
CPT code that describes the ingrown nail as painful or in-
fected. Otherwise the insurance company with think that the
procedure is "cosmetic" (seriously!) and will not cover the cost.
(Since when did having your toenails ripped off become a cosmetic procedure like having your face lifted? Ugh! You won't
see me having this "cosmetic" procedure done anytime soon. I
like having toenails, thank you.)

International Statistical Classification of Diseases and
Related Health Problem codes, or ICD codes for short, were
formulated back in 1900 as a way to classify diseases, signs
and symptoms, and general abnormal findings. Every health

condition has an ICD code. We are currently using the ninth revision of the coding system, which was published in 1977 (making it archaic by now) and has 17,000 different codes. The ICD-10 revision was completed in 1992 and has more than 155,000 codes. The United States has not yet adopted ICD-10 codes and is still using the limited ICD-9 codes, which is likely an advantage for the insurance companies. ICD-9 codes, therefore, add a new level of complexity to the billing and coding language that exists among hospital, doctors, and payers. After a while this numeric language becomes incomprehensible gibberish, which the insurance companies use as a reason not to pay. Keep in mind that the game the insurance companies are playing is to try to find ways in which they don't have to pay doctors and hospitals (one of my coders refers to insurance companies as "professional thieves"). If we submit a code that is off by a single number, they don't pay. If we submit an ICD-9 code that doesn't "work" with a particular CPT code, they don't pay. If the bill gets to the insurance company late, they don't pay. If we don't respond to a billing inquiry within a narrow time frame (insurance companies are notorious for postdating their inquiry letters to narrow the response time frame to just a few days), they don't pay. If you have blue eyes, they don't pay. So don't gasp the next time you see your hospital bill. We doctors will never, *never ever*, see the dollars posted on your bill.

Do you know how much I received for Dan's eleven-hour case, which, by the way, does not include the hours I spent at his bedside taking care of him, my 24/7 availability for any and all calls about him from the hospital staff or his family, and the time spent during his follow-up visits to my office? About

$3,000. For our most routine case, a triple-bypass surgery, we receive approximately $1,700 to $2,000. As an assisting surgeon, you receive 16 percent of what the CPT code pays, which is a few hundred bucks. The CPT code for an endoscopic vein harvest, which is cosmetically and functionally better for the patient and ultimately less painful than opening the entire leg, pays $15.09!

Now let me put this in perspective for you. I get paid $3,000 for eleven-plus hours of work that includes shutting down the human heart and then bringing it back, not to mention the seventeen years of school and training it took to be able to do that. This equates to $272 an hour. If we account for all of my other time taking care of Dan after his surgery, we're probably down to less than $30 an hour. My hairdresser, Nathan (whom I love dearly), gets a $5,000 day rate for going to the home of a *Sex and the City* actress and doing a cut and blow-dry. He also tells me that this is "cheap" by Hollywood standards.

So what's the message here? The message here is that people are valued differently for their jobs, and if you are a cardiac surgeon who is in it only for the money, you won't be in it for long. It's not about the money. It's about the thrill of touching the human heart. It's about the passion you have for getting up every morning and knowing that today you will help a complete stranger. It's about going to bed exhausted from the healing that you've done all day.

But, of course, a surgeon has to eat. A surgeon has to have a roof over her head. A surgeon, like everyone else, wants to give her children a better educational opportunity than she had (I had never heard of an AP credit until I showed up at college without any) at a school where gun control isn't the board's main budgetary concern. I pride myself in the fact that, in addition to my husband, I am also a breadwinner for my family. Earning an honest living is important to me.

• • •

I am very worried about the future of cardiac surgery. First and foremost, fewer and fewer residents are going into my field; in fact, we haven't been able to fill the number of cardiothoracic training spots available in the United States for the last several years. According to the most recent data, one third of the training spots remained unfilled.* It takes a long time to train and so you defer income for a longer period in the face of mounting debt from student loans. I am still, at the age of forty-five, paying off a student loan! When you do finish, the income you receive for your long, complicated, risky work is far less than it used to be thanks to reimbursement by insurance companies that seriously do not understand how to value a doctor's efforts. Especially when the orthopedic back surgeon who did Dan's back surgery four months later made $4,000 for a two-hour low-risk case with minimal postoperative care. Dan was in the hospital for over a week after his eleven-hour heart surgery procedure and went home two days after his back surgery.

Medical students and residents know this when they are making their career choices in medicine. For the same reasons, we are now looking at a profound shortage of internists and family practice doctors as well. In a *USA Today* article, the number of medical students going into primary care has dropped 52 percent since 1997, putting the current doctor-to-

*Grover, Atul, et al., "Shortage of cardiothoracic surgeons is likely by 2020," *Circulation* (2009) 120:488–94.

patient ratio at 400 to 1.* Students are simply choosing more lucrative specialties. But it's not just about the paucity of income relative to other less demanding jobs. The lifestyle of a cardiac surgeon is rough. I am essentially on call and reachable at all times. Not only that, but because of the life I chose, I had to defer marriage and children. Most female medical students and undergrads whom I speak with feel it is simply *impossible* to be a married heart surgeon with kids, and for that reason they seek "women-friendly" specialties. The few women who eventually do choose cardiothoracic surgery end up doing only thoracic (lung) surgery because there are no middle-of-the-night emergency lung cancer resections, and so the lifestyle is better. Currently only 3 percent of cardiothoracic surgeons are women.[†] Thus, there are fewer and fewer "cardiac chicks" like me.

I am also sincerely worried about the surgical caseload in cardiac surgery. With the introduction of statin drugs, to prevent coronary artery disease, and stents, which allow interventional cardiologists to treat coronary artery disease in a less invasive manner, cardiac surgeons have seen a sharp decline in coronary artery bypass grafting (CABG) cases. According to a recent article, CABG surgeries, which are our bread-and-butter surgeries, have declined between 14.1 percent (all insured patients) and 22.3 percent (Medicare-insured patients) from 2001 to 2005.[‡] Cardiac surgeons have had to rely on heart valve procedures to make up for this CABG volume loss.

*USA Today, August 21, 2009, section 8A.
[†]Grover, Atul, et al., "Shortage of cardiothoracic surgeons is likely by 2020."
[‡]James L. Field, MBA, DBA, "Current and future market trends in cardiothoracic surgery," *Society of Thoracic Surgeons STS News*, 14, no. S1 (July 2008): 1–6.

However, new technology currently in clinical trial allows cardiologists to replace heart valves percutaneously. Two companies, Edwards Lifescience and Medtronic, are in competition to perfect two new valves that can be implanted through catheters. Similar to a cardiac catheterization, this would be a minimally invasive procedure that does not require the chest to be opened. These valves have been available in Europe for the past eighteen months and are in clinical trials in the United States. Between statins, stents, and percutaneous valves, what will heart surgeons do for a living? The new percutaneous valves will cost approximately $30,000 whereas the valves that I implant surgically cost $5,000. Maybe the "fiscally responsible" insurance companies will side with us cardiothoracic surgeons on this one. (Don't hold your breath.)

It is imperative that the cardiac surgeon evolve by using cutting-edge techniques that minimize the invasiveness of operations. Otherwise we will become obsolete. If history is any indication of our fate, however, we will evolve and survive. When tuberculosis first became an epidemic, it was treated only by surgery, and thus thoracic surgery was born. In the wake of antibiotics discovered in 1944, there was a sharp decline in thoracic surgery until, eventually, surgery was rarely used to treat TB. The eradication of TB forced thoracic surgeons to evolve into lung cancer and esophagus surgeons who remain working to this day.

It is also imperative that we evolve by being better team players. For far too long we have been the lone wolves in the tundra of cardiovascular disease. It is time for us to join forces with our colleagues who also work in the realm of cardiovascular disease, rather than see them as competition. I am not just talking about cardiologists, although that is a likely partnership. I am more interested in seeing joint ventures with invasive radiologists and vascular surgeons. We are at least starting down this road. Hospitals are creating "cardiovascular institutes" within their medical centers that provide a multidisciplinary approach to heart disease. In these institutes, heart surgeons work in hybrid ORs with radiologists and vascular surgeons to implant large stents within the aorta to treat an aortic aneurysm (an abnormal enlargement of the aorta) or even an aortic dissection. We can also utilize the hybrid OR to work with interventional cardiologists to perform minimally invasive bypass surgery or combined procedures with coronary artery stenting. These ORs are a combination of a full surgical suite complete with a heart-lung machine, a state-of-the-art cardiac catheterization lab, and a sophisticated radiology suite. Hybrid ORs allow us to jointly perform minimally invasive cardiovascular procedures with the safety net of being able to immediately convert to an open procedure if necessary.

Another testament to the "join or die" idea is the fact that many cardiothoracic surgery training programs are now requiring the residents to spend a portion of their training in the cardiac catheterization lab working with a cardiologist to learn this skill set. During my training, we didn't dare set foot in the cath lab unless specifically called to do so.

But it's not all doom and gloom yet for us cardiac surgeons. There are still some nasty types of heart disease that continue to increase in prevalence and for which there is no truly curative medical therapy. Congestive heart failure is a prime example. CHF affects 4.8 million Americans and the number of cases continues to be on the rise, with approximately 400,000 new cases yearly. It is the leading diagnosis in 875,000 hospitalizations and is the most common admitting diagnosis in the United States in patients sixty-five years and older. CHF is responsible for one-fifth of all hospitalizations.

Once diagnosed with CHF, half of all patients will die within five years. Surgical treatments such as bypass grafting, valve repair or replacement, stem cell therapy (experimental), ventricular assist device placement, and heart transplantation still remain the best option for most patients who are candidates for such procedures.

Of course, there is also heart disease in women to fall back on . . .

Please don't misunderstand me. I don't want people to smoke cigarettes and eat foie gras just so I can stay in business. On the contrary. I would like to see heart disease eradicated. But still today, as you read this, men and women are dying in epidemic proportions and there is still so much good that I can do. But really, the problem is bigger than just the dilemma facing cardiac surgery. We are just a stubbed toe on the foot of a much greater problem.

If we step back and look at the larger picture for a moment, you will see that it is not just cardiac surgeons who are an endangered species but the whole of health care as we know it. I am uncertain that the health care system, in its current state, can survive much longer. It is such a shame, really, that no one can figure out what is wrong when the problem is very simple. It's just a broken equation that we are dealing with. A very simple, broken equation: Profit = Revenue – Cost, where Revenue = Price × Quantity. Hospitals, the pillars that hold up the health care system, are becoming unstable because of this equation, and when they are unstable, health care is unstable. When they fall, health care in this country will fall. Despite cost-cutting measures, hospitals cannot stabilize financially because of price constraints. The "price" that a hospital commands is the equivalent of what insurers will pay. If you were to go into a Gap store and pick up a T-shirt that costs $15, bring it to the checkout counter, and put down a $5 bill, would you be able to walk out with that T-shirt? No. Ned's insurance company was billed approximately $385,000 for his heart surgery hospitalization. The insurance company paid the hospital $54,000, or approximately 14 percent of the bill, and, believe me, a hospital is ecstatic whenever it collects more than 10 percent of the bill. How can hospitals not only survive but be expected to deliver state-of-the-art care when their price is not met? They can only increase their quantity until the hospital is full. They can only cut their costs until the delivery of quality health care is jeopardized. This is why hospitals turn away the uninsured. They have no margin to take on this debt. Ten million people reside in Los Angeles County and there are eighty-seven hospitals to take care of these people. Over the past decade, fourteen hospitals in LA have closed owing to financial hardship. Of these eighty-seven remaining hospitals, only thirty-four have positive operating margins; the rest are operating in the negative.

If the insurance companies would simply pay what they are billed rather than just choosing to pay whatever they feel like paying, the health care system will stabilize and there will be plenty for all. The answer is not simply giving everyone health insurance, although that may represent a partial solution. The answer is for the insurance companies to take responsibility and to pay the hospital what they bill, as is the practice of any business entity.

Now don't even get me started about how lawyers are driving up health care costs because we are forced to practice defensive medicine . . .

• • •

The way that I have chosen to evolve as a cardiac surgeon is to increase the number of arrows in my quiver, which is, I guess, why I ultimately pursued an MBA. I knew I was in over my head, however, when I hooked my first finance exam ("hooked" being slang for getting a C). Actually, I failed the exam and then rode the curve up to a C. The only people who passed on their own merit were the chief financial officers in the class. Who am I to compete with them? Now, if there had been more questions about the aorta on the exam, I might have passed, but quite honestly, the whole course blew me away.

I thought that medical school had been tough, but attending the UCLA Anderson School of Management was an entirely different game on an entirely different playing field. I am often asked, "Why the MBA?" I suppose it was simply that I wanted to broaden my educational horizon. I was forty-one years old and had been doing nothing but cardiac surgery for the past six years. It's not that I wanted to give up being a surgeon; I just wanted to expand my palette. The business world and the world of medicine often collide in an unnatural way when, in fact, they should be intertwined in a working relationship. Like it or not, medicine *is* a business just like Walmart or FedEx. It's just one of the most poorly run businesses you've ever seen.

In the past, I had worked with medical technology companies to help them develop cardiac devices that would save lives. I could only function as a clinical consultant, helping them to develop the device so that it fit properly in the human body and functioned well in clinical circumstances. What I found, though, was that these companies really needed help with bringing their product to market, in other words, crossing the chasm between developing their product and actually getting it to the patients who need it most. But I was at a loss to help them with things like building a business plan, doing a market analysis, and procuring venture capital funding, because I couldn't speak the language of business. If I could do both—help them clinically and strategically—then perhaps, indirectly, I could save more lives than just the one or two patients I operate on each day.

The other reason for going to business school was more selfish. I simply wanted to use my brain again. I was in my forties, had just had a child, and was doing a job that was more technical than intellectual. It had been decades since I had sat in a classroom and learned something new. Decades since I had taken an exam. Decades since I had written a paper. I guess I just wanted to feed my brain again and feel intellectually stimulated. Of course, it helped that I had had a life-altering lunch with a brilliant, successful, poised businesswoman, Larraine, who looked across the table at me when I was complaining about my doldrums and said, point-blank, "You know what you need? You need an MBA!" God love the woman, because with her encouragement, that's exactly what I did.

I now have an MBA and am utilizing it to build a business model for a women's health center at my hospital. I have also, along with two brilliant colleagues, recently patented a medical device that is a noninvasive, nonimaging device that can reliably predict the early onset of heart disease. We are in the process of simplifying and testing our latest prototype and our LLC is called Cordex Systems.

So, sure, I failed the finance exam, but I certainly did love the challenge! Always have, always will. The lesson here is that it's never too late to reinvent yourself. Especially if, in your unforeseeable future, it helps you to evolve.

17

Atypical Weekend

W HAT MAY SEEM LIKE AN ATYPICAL WEEKEND FOR YOU is quite a typical weekend for me, I can assure you. The first thing you need to know about my weekends is that there are no such things as weekends. Saturday and Sunday don't exist as nonworking days for me. To me, Saturday and Sunday just mean that I get to park a little closer to the hospital. So on Monday morning, please don't ask me about my "weekend" or, on Friday, ask me, "Kathy, what are you doing this week-end?" Just treat it like any other day. My job is 24/7. If I am in town, then I am available. The only way for me to be "off call" is to be in Tibet or dead.

The other thing you need to know about my weekends is that there is no "sleeping in." This begins with no full night's sleep and culminates with the inevitable 6:00 a.m. phone call from the ICU to update me on all of the patients prior to the nurse's change of shift at 7:00 a.m. My husband has all of his calls forwarded to our home number—and so the bedside phone rings all night long. I can be reached by cell, pager, or home number, and the nurses randomly choose which form of communication they wish to use. In a dire emergency they use all three—simultaneously. This means that throughout the night there is a free jazz symphony of harsh ring tones that sound not unlike a calliope. Similar to a mother who can discern the cry of her own baby, I am in tune with my own ring tones and can (almost) sleep through some of Nick's calls. When guests stay overnight at our house, they awaken the next morning with that bleary look that says, "Did you hear the phones ringing all night long?" Hey, I never said that the Nissen-Magliato Hotel guarantees a full night's sleep. After all, we're not a Holiday Inn Express.

When the calls at night involve something minor like "Give ten milli-equivalents of potassium" or "Start amiodarone," I can usually roll over and fall back to sleep quickly. When the call involves a more complicated problem that requires coherent thought, whoever gets the call sits up in bed and talks through the problem with the caller. This awakens the other person in bed and, now that we're both up, we usually discuss the problem at hand, liver, pancreas, or heart, and the treatment plan. Nick and I have had some of our best conversations in the dead of night. We even take the opportunity to ask how the other is doing, or to find out how the workday was, or to put together a to-do list for the house, or discuss the latest developments in the saga of getting our five-year-old into kindergarten. We like to bounce things off each other in the middle of the night because we never know when we will have the opportunity to talk again.

My husband is usually called about potential liver donors in the wee hours of the night, which forces me to hear about a nine-year-old boy who came home from school with a headache and went on to die from meningitis. I can honestly tell you that after hearing information like this, there is no more sleep for me. Sometimes the calls are life or death. You just never know. The call usually takes the form of a very curt one-liner from a breathless nurse: "Your patient [no name given, leaving you to search your mind for who is your sickest patient and most likely to die] just arrested" or "Your patient just dumped seven hundred cc's from their chest tubes [in my case] or abdominal drains [in my husband's case]." Either way, it translates to "They're bleeding to death." That's when all hell breaks loose in a typical night at my house. Before the nurse can even get to the word *arrested* or *dumped,* our feet are already on the ground. By the time the nurse utters the definitive verb we are running to find the scrubs that we keep, for efficiency's sake, on the floor next to our bed along with our sneakers and keys. Can you imagine having to bolt out of your bed at two o'clock on a Saturday morning, get dressed, get in your car, and speed to the hospital with your flashers on while trying to avoid the drunks who are invariably on the road in LA at that hour? You then need to be completely awake and alert by the time you arrive at the hospital to face the challenge that awaits you. All the while you're hoping that no one notices that you have "morning breath" or are wearing no makeup. If I took the time to brush my teeth or apply a little mascara, someone could die. Imagine that. A life hangs in the balance over mere seconds of personal hygiene.

Now that I have clearly established that I don't sleep through my typical weekend night, please allow me to elaborate on why there is no sleeping in on weekends. This is because when I get my "change-of-shift" call at 6:00 a.m., this

wakes up both of my children, who, at the ages of three and
five, are in the lightest phases of their sleep cycle at that hour.
Our children don't know that a weekend is any different from
any other day of the week, since we work every day, and so I
hear their bedroom door open and the pitter-pat of feet on
the wood floor in the hallway that adjoins our rooms. I usually try to pretend that I am asleep when they get to our
room, but inevitably I cannot hold a sleeping pose, especially
when they put their little faces close to mine and proclaim,
"Mommy, it's a new day!" They say this every morning without fail and it is a wonderful beginning. No matter how bad
a night my husband and I had—even with the sickest of patients, or after listening to the tragedy of a young donor—we
always begin the next day with two boys announcing "It's a
new day." That one line changes everything. It washes away
the distress of the night before. It is a cleansing breath. For a
new day has come, and in the eyes of these children, it is a
day of hope and wonderment.

   The last thing that you need to know about my weekend
is that I always have one minor secret personal goal to accomplish. It's usually to get a manicure (no nail polish, just
buffed) and a pedicure (with some goth color like Russian
Navy by Opi). Shh. Don't tell anybody. I need to sneak off to
do this so that my kids and my husband don't know. No one
knows. I usually do it under the guise of having to go in and
make rounds. "Yeah, honey, rounds took longer than I thought,"
I say, trying to hide my blue toes, which just this morning
were bright red. He never notices. Must be a guy thing. I
mean, don't you think it's a little obvious that I am arriving
home from the hospital in flip-flops? I know it's selfish, but
can't I have just this one thing? I try to justify it by saying to

myself that since I am a surgeon and my hands are my tools, I need to take care of them. Clean, short nails. Trim cuticles. Haven't been able to justify the pedi, though. I go to great lengths for this one indulgence. I schedule my rounds around when I can get an available appointment. I factor the toenail polish drying time into the equation and hope that it results in a successful formula.

So let's take a look at last weekend, because it represents a fairly typical one for me. What I immediately noticed about my impending weekend being on first-call was that it landed on a full moon in the lunar phase cycle. Ask any doctor—a full moon weekend brings with it universal insanity. The hospital is usually chaotic and busy. The ED is a sandstorm of people. Lots of admissions. Crazy things happen. There is a very real and palpable change in the hospital atmosphere. A colleague will stop you in the hall and ask, "Is there a full moon or what?" to which you reply, "Feels like it."

As if that weren't bad enough, Nick was also on first-call, which meant he was taking all the hits, too. There are usually two surgeons on call on any given day. The first-call surgeon handles all of the admissions, performs emergency surgery if needed, and takes all of the phone calls from any inpatient or outpatient of anyone in the surgical group. The first-call surgeon also makes hospital rounds on all of their own patients and their partners' patients. This entails seeing and examining each patient; discussing the treatment plan with the patient, their family, and their nurse; checking every patient's laboratory values and every X-ray or other such study they have had; and writing a comprehensive note in every patient's chart. In other words, when you are on first-call, you do the brunt of the work. If you are at a teaching hospital, as is my husband, then there are interns and residents who can look up the relevant data on the patients and facilitate rounds. If you are at a nonteaching hospital, as I am, then YOYO (you're on your own). Rounds take longer but—and here's the trade-off—I am responsible only for my own work. Second-call is a better call position because you only need to come in if the first-call surgeon needs help with a surgical case that has presented itself over the weekend. You still have to be sober and be near the medical center, so you can't really run amok on second-call. If you practice at a transplant center, then there may even be a third-call surgeon, whose job it is to go out on a donor organ procurement for a transplant. So last weekend, not only were Nick and I both on first-call, but, our caregiver had the weekend off. This is considered a trifecta in our work-family balance and a recipe for disaster.

My best friend and heart disease survivor, Donna, had invited Nick and me over for a Saturday-afternoon dinner party (notice I didn't say "weekend"). Although the occasion was meant to be casual, I saw the opportunity to wear my new Michael Kors black platform sandals (with chunky five-inch cork heels), which I had picked up at Bergdorf's the last time I was in New York City. I wanted to show them off to Donna, an avid shoe collector. I showed up with my heels, my husband, and my kids in tow, and just as I was striding (with the perfect balance and precision becoming of a surgeon) up her uneven brick walkway, my pager goes off. It's the ED and that's a bad sign.

"I got a guy in the ED here who dropped his right lung. It's one hundred percent down. The X-ray is very cool looking. He's satting [doctor-speak for 'saturating,' meaning the oxygen level in his blood] well on a mask. A little tacky, though. The guy's talking to me. Pretty amazing. Listen, I'm too busy to put a chest tube in him; can you come and stick one in? If he goes south, I'll poke him with a needle." This is the narrative that I heard on my cell phone from the ED physician. I don't know which was more disturbing to me: the fact that the patient was tachycardic ("tacky"), meaning his heart rate was elevated, or the fact that I wasn't sure if the doctor on the other end of the phone understood the profound significance of this seemingly trivial piece of information.

When I was a kid, Nana, my mother's mother, had this uncanny ability to look down upon a bed of clover in the side yard between her house and ours and within a few seconds pluck a four-leaf clover from among the thousands of three-leaf clover leaves in the bed. I, on the other hand, would spend hours in the yard looking for this small treasure among the four-leaf-clover wannabes. That is, until I developed her knack for it. When someone is presenting a critically ill patient to me, like this one, I home in on the lethal detail, which is often hidden and small. It's a gift my nana gave me.

This patient had what we refer to as a complete spontaneous tension pneumothorax. It means that his lung has spontaneously deflated, and as a result of a pressure buildup in his thoracic cavity, his heart and the great vessels supplying blood to it have shifted in the direction opposite the side of the pneumothorax. This shift causes a kinking of these vessels and results in death owing to a profound decrease of blood flow entering the heart. The first sign that this kinking is starting to occur is an elevated heart rate. The next sign is a profound drop in blood pressure and the next sign is a full-on cardiac arrest.

We usually see a spontaneous pneumothorax in young,

thin males who have no underlying lung disease per se but rupture a bleb at the top or apical area of a lung. A bleb is a small (less than one centimeter) airspace just beneath the lining of the lung known as the pleura. Older patients can get a pneumothorax as a result of having emphysema. They often rupture a bulla, which is a large thinned-out portion of the lung. People with lung cancer, asthma, connective tissue disorders, endometriosis, or a lung infection can blow a hole in a lung and cause it to deflate. Trauma to the chest can do this as well.

I quickly say hello to Donna, dump the kids in Nick's arms, and say to no particular person, "Someone's trying to die. Gotta go." Donna kisses me good-bye and says, "You go save a life, honey. We'll see you back here later for dinner." The last thing I hear her say is "You're not going to go into the hospital in those! Do you want some sensible shoes [like she has any]? You'll ruin those." Too late, I was already in my car and backing out of her driveway.

I was at the hospital in minutes. I checked the chest X-ray to make sure the diagnosis was correct and that the right side was indeed the side where the chest tube was needed. Trust no one. I always double-check *everything* lest one cuts off the wrong leg or takes out the wrong testicle (both of which have been done). Incidentally, this has a name—it's called wrong-site surgery. To prevent this, we now give patients a Sharpie maker in the preoperative holding room and have them mark the site of the surgery. It gives them a little artistic license as well.

I went into the patient's room in the ED and found him just as he was described—sitting up on a gurney looking a little pale and short of breath. He was wearing an oxygen mask, and although his oxygen saturation was acceptable ("he's satting well"), his heart rate was climbing and his blood pressure dipping a bit. He was surprisingly alert and even jovial. Because he could crash at any minute, I kept one eye on his vital signs while I calmly and pleasantly spoke with him. If he were to crash, I knew I could save him by sticking a large 14-gauge needle directly into the front of his right chest about three fingerbreadths below his collarbone and in line with his nipple. This maneuver relieves the air under pressure that has built up in his chest; it is similar to popping a balloon. I had managed to sneak a 14-gauge needle into my white-coat pocket on my way to his room for just such an occasion. I was armed but not dangerous.

While I am setting up the instrument tray that I will use to put in the chest tube, I engage him in conversation to distract him from what I am about to do and hopefully make him more at ease with me. "What do you do?" I asked. "I invent designer hallucinogenic drugs," he replied.

"You're kidding. Really? How?" I'm intrigued.

"I take a known hallucinogenic that's a bit of an upper and put a methyl group on it. It makes the drug less edgy and jittery," he said.

"A true connoisseur," I thought. It turns out he had a PhD in chemistry and an MBA from a top-ten business school. Being a biochemistry major, I tried to call his bluff by having him draw the molecular structure of a popular clubbing drug. He drew it, pointed out the methyl group, and explained the entire chemical formula to me. I meet all kinds of people in my line of work.

When I finish prepping his chest, I inject lidocaine (similar to novocaine, which a dentist uses) to numb any pain sensation he might feel in the area in which I am working. I make a small incision in his right side, where I will put the chest tube into his thoracic cavity. The chest tube is a fifteen-inch-long firm plastic tube that comes in different diameters ranging from the diameter of a pencil to the diameter of a quarter. I locate the space between two ribs where I will poke a hole into his chest with a blunt hemostat. As I am about to apply pressure to the hemostat and enter this man's chest, my cell phone rings and the ED nurse who is in the room with me answers it. "It's Donna," she says. "She wants you to know that the brisket will be ready in thirty minutes." In that instant the patient and I are reminded that life goes on out there beyond what we are about to do here in this ED. The patient turns to me and with a rather charming, wry smile repeats, "The brisket will be ready in thirty minutes," and with that, I plunge the hemostat deftly into his chest. There is a huge rush of air that escapes his chest. His heart rate comes down. His blood pressure goes up. Still smiling, he says that he can breathe much better now. And just like that I saved this man, a complete stranger. Nothing in life could be more rewarding.

The last thing he said to me as I left the ER to join the dinner party was "Nice shoes." That's when I looked down and realized that I had just slammed a chest tube in while wearing five-inch heels and managed not to get a drop of blood on them. Pretty slick.

The next day of my so-called weekend (aka Sunday) required Nick and me to do a little planning that we call our rounding strategy. This is a discussion that we have to see who gets to go in first and make rounds on all the patients when we are both on first-call. We do this so that one of us can be home with the children. We usually use the rule of thumb that whoever has the most or sickest patients wins, and that person gets to do rounds first. The problem with these two rules is that Nick usually wins. Now recall, if you will, that I have an ulterior motive at play here—to get a mani-pedi. I therefore make a good argument for how my patients are sicker than his and get to go in first. With my mani-pedi scheduled for noon, I should have plenty of time to get rounds done and get to my appointment. I make my rounds and all is going well. A little too well for a full-moon weekend. I am suspicious.

I get a call just after arriving at the hospital from the cardiac catheterization lab that one of the cardiologists is doing a cath and wants me to "take a look at the films." This means he wants me to see the results of the catheterization while the patient is still on the procedure table and render a surgical opinion. I head down to the cath lab, look at the patient's film, and discuss it with the cardiologist who did the case. He and I are in agreement that the patient would best benefit from open heart surgery to bypass the blockages that he found in the patient's coronary arteries as opposed to treating him with angioplasty and stenting. He tells me the patient is young and relatively healthy except for having high blood pressure. What he neglects to tell me, however, is that the patient is profoundly bipolar (manic-depressive) and has been off his psychiatric medication for three days.

I decide that because the patient was given a light sedation for the cardiac catheterization, I will finish my rounds and see him just before I leave the hospital so that the sedation can wear off and he and I can have a coherent discussion about his impending operation. I finish my rounds and get to his bedside at 11:00 a.m. I introduce myself and begin to take his history, asking him about what brought him to the hospital. He seems like a nice enough guy but is clearly manic. His speech is pressured and he gestures wildly. After taking his history, I begin my exam. As I approach closer to listen to his heart and lungs with my stethoscope, he suddenly pulls out a knife that he had hidden in his bed. He starts waving it wildly at me just inches from my face while saying, "Look at my knife! Look at my knife! Isn't it a beauty?" Without flinching, because I didn't want him to sense fear, I calmly and with feigned exuberance exclaimed, "Wow! That is a *really* great knife! You know I'm a surgeon and just *love* knives! Gee, do you think I could hold it?" He hands it to me and I abruptly turn away from him and leave the room with it stowed in my pocket. His nurse, Kristen, is waiting outside the room. "Whaddyawanna do with the knife?" she asks. "Call security," I say. "What a crazy few days. Yesterday I put a chest tube in a guy who makes club drugs and today I get a knife pulled on me." "Must be a full moon," Kristen responds. To which I reply, "Feels like it."

As I leave the hospital I look down at my watch. It's 1:00 p.m.

Damn!

I missed my noon nail appointment.

Again.

18

Kids Are Alright

USED TO TEST MYSELF TO SEE IF I WANTED TO HAVE KIDS by strolling down the cereal aisle at the local grocery store. There I'd inevitably find a mom with a screaming child in her arms and another crying child in the grocery cart, one leg over the side, trying desperately to take a header to the floor. It made it easier for me that I had a demanding career that squeezed all thought of having kids completely out of my head. But then a special man, your soul mate, blows into your life and change is in the wind . . .

• • •

She stirred just once, turned her head to the right so that it gently rested against my chest and then was still. Abnormally still. More still than a baby should lie even in the deepest of slumbers. She died with no name. She died without her parents present. But at least she died while being cradled in someone's arms—my own.

She was eleven days old and I had spent every moment of her eleven days on this earth at her bedside trying desperately to save her. She was born with a large hole in her heart called an atrioventricular canal, or AV canal for short. When I think of canals, I think of beautiful waterways in Venice filled with romance and adventure. This canal of the heart was in no way similar to the Venetian form of transit. This one was filled with death. Blue babies floating in it deprived of oxygen while their blood intermingled between chambers.

Her parents, fearing she might not survive, did not name her. As if, somehow, they would be less likely to become attached to her. By not naming her, there was no ownership. The signage on her incubator read simply BABY GIRL. The nurses had named her Elizabeth, which, coincidentally, is my middle name and also my mom's middle name and was the name of both my grandmothers.

At the time, I was in my first of two years of residency training in cardiothoracic surgery. I spent a terrifying six months on the pediatric service, where we operated on the sickest of the sick—children with congenital heart disease. Forty thousand infants are born each year with heart disease, which equates to one out of every thousand births. Twice as many children die of congenital heart disease than from all forms of childhood cancers combined. They are the "blue babies" one often hears about. So named because of the bluish hue of unoxygenated blood circulating through their bodies. This is also known as cyanosis.

My job was to keep babies alive after they underwent long, complicated operations, the likes of which would kill the average adult. Caring for these infants was one of the most difficult tasks in my residency training. Every budding cardiothoracic surgeon fears this pediatric rotation because it is, by far, the most demanding. At this particular hospital, however, we also feared the rotation because if a kid died on your watch, the attending pediatric cardiothoracic surgeon, a short, malignant guy, would point to you in the middle of the neonatal ICU and yell loudly for all to hear, "YOU [*he would pause for emphasis*] KILLED THE BABY!" This would inevitably blow a hole right through my chest every time. What made things worse was that these infants were incredibly difficult to manage because their precarious postoperative condition is in a constant state of flux requiring minute-to-minute adjustments in their treatment. Even the smallest mistake in judgment can kill them.

They are, however, remarkably resilient. They are the fighters. You think they cannot possibly stand such long, arduous procedures. You think they will surely die. And they, the little fighters, fool you every time.

The funny thing was, I thought Elizabeth was going to live. I was wrong. Fooled again. When she died, she took a little piece of me with her, like flesh torn away from the bone.

And so I found myself perched at this little girl's bedside for eleven straight days (my personal in-house record) following the surgery to close the hole in her heart. I never left the hospital. Meals were few and far between. What little sleep I got was in a rocking chair at her bedside. These chairs were used for lactating mothers who were allowed to remove their babies from their incubators and nurse them. For me, the rocking chair was my post. My camp. From the vantage point of that chair I gave the orders to the nurses to adjust Elizabeth's medications in an effort to save her life, to win a grave battle. The more medication I ordered, the more we had to fall back on when she didn't respond. Not a full retreat, mind you, because that would be giving up and I *never* give up, no matter how fierce the battle. Unless, of course, it is the family's wish.

In the end, it was her parents who gave up the fight. All it took was one word: "Enough." Not "enough" as in, "You've tried enough," because that would have eased my burden. They meant "enough" as in, "She's had enough." As if I had flogged this little girl into existence on a daily basis for the past eleven days. This only made my burden, my pain, heavier. I suspect, however, that, in part, they meant, too, "enough" as in, "*We've* had enough." They were tired. They were exhausted physically and emotionally. And, unknowingly perhaps, they gave up the one weapon that can win or lose a battle for life—hope. Hope is so powerful that it can overcome the greatest of enemies, which is fear. The only other weapon we have that rivals hope is the will to live.

Respecting their wishes, we quietly disconnected all of Elizabeth's tubes and lines. It was a very somber moment. The nurses, their faces emotionless, did this in a methodical manner as if they had disconnected babies from life support a thousand times. Maybe they had. Maybe this was a dance of death that was already so well choreographed it made it all the easier to perform. How was I to know? I was a young cardiothoracic trainee and had never seen a child taken off life support before. Each intravenous medication was slowly turned off. Each monitor disconnected. It was quiet now. Very, very quiet. A hush came over the area around her incubator as if silencing an audience when a play is about to begin.

The parents were waiting in a little room down the hall where they could neither see nor hear what we were doing. They retreated and I could not blame them. The horror of losing a child is a cut that runs deep. It can be lethal to the parents and they need to survive so that there may be other children for them in the future.

Where was I during all of this? In my rocking chair at Elizabeth's bedside, of course. Ever at my post. The nurses then did something that I will never forget. After Elizabeth was disconnected, they reached into the incubator, drew her out, and gently handed her to me. I was thirty-four years old and, not having held many children, was awkwardly holding this baby. Like trying to hold a seven-pound bag of marbles, I kept shifting her weight in my arms.

The pain was unbearable. I felt my heart break in two. I could hardly look at her there in my arms as I fought back tears. In my head I kept saying, "Don't cry! Don't cry! You'll look weak. You have to be stronger than that!" Why? Why do I have to be stronger than that? Why can't I just cry? Why do I have to just let her go as if her death doesn't affect me in the slightest? Why can't I just let the pain wash over me and cleave me in two? Why must I feel nothing and be completely shielded from the sting of death in my nostrils, blood in my eye, failure in my marrow? If I feel nothing, then I can wander at will, for the rest of my career, through the stale, dank corridors of the hospital awash in sickness and frailty and I will be untouchable. I will be unscathed. I will be invincible. I will be invisible. A ghost among the wreckage of lives seeing everything and feeling nothing.

But right then and there I made a choice. A choice that forever changed me. I chose to feel it all and not let it go. I chose to find dignity, compassion, and kindness in this sweet child's death. I chose to hold her when she took her last little breath and not turn away.

When she died a few moments later, her little body seemed to get lighter. Was her soul released? Holding her became neither difficult nor awkward. She was a bag of feathers.

I then took the most difficult walk that I have ever taken. Many walks in my life have been difficult and fearful—when I walked into my first class in medical school, when I walked into my first patient's room, when I walked into my first operation. This walk—down the hallway to the parents' room while carrying their dead baby—was filled with a mixture of compassion and pain. Not failure. Not fear.

As I approached the parents' room, I kissed Elizabeth on her forehead. Her skin was cool and soft and she still had that "new baby" smell that all parents recognize. I handed the dead baby girl to her mother without making eye contact, something I have always regretted. I couldn't look at her. She would see my pain. My vulnerability.

Without a word, I turned and left the room, left the hospital immediately. I didn't speak to anyone on my way out. Eyes down, bent with exhaustion. I was finally free of it all. I could exhale. I could run away. I could feel the wind again, a breeze in my life that would blow away the staleness of death that clung to me. I went home to my apartment, where I could be alone in a place of sanctuary to heal. I needed to regroup so that I could join the battle again tomorrow.

I mistakenly thought that tomorrow would somehow be better than the previous day. How could it be worse? Conjoined twins, that's how.

. . .

The first page I received that morning was from my boss, the malignant pediatric cardiac surgeon. He wanted me to come up to the "unit" (the neonatal ICU) ASAP for a "complex and interesting" consult. When I arrived, I couldn't find the attending. I asked a nurse where Dr. Ponce was, and she answered, "Behind the screen, over there," pointing to the farthermost section of the unit. A white screen had been set up around an incubator. When I came around the side of the screen, all I could see was a large baby who looked like he or she had its hand in the air. When I got a better look, I saw a child with two heads and one very wide body with an arm on each side where they naturally exist. There was a third arm, however, coming from behind and between the two heads that was pointing upward. The legs were covered in a blanket but I could tell there were more than two. A young woman with no prenatal care had delivered the children a few hours earlier. We had been consulted to see if the children could be separated based on the cardiac morphology. Unfortunately, an echocardiogram showed that these Siamese twins shared a common heart from which they could not be separated. Their blood intermingled, forever bonded as one. The parents decided to take their babies home and I have no idea whatever happened to them.

That was it for me. No kids. I swore off kids. Throughout my years of training I was asked incessantly in the OR by male surgeons, "When are you going to find a guy? When are you going to get married? When are you going to have kids?" to which I flatly answered, "Never. Never. And never." Besides, it was none of their business, but "never" is a really long time . . .

• • •

The first thing I noticed was that my husband's shoulders were rhythmically moving up and down in a jerky motion. Nick had his back to me, and because I couldn't see his face, I thought he was laughing. But suddenly two things struck me at once: I hadn't heard the baby cry yet, and oh my God, Nick was crying, not laughing. His shoulders were moving that way because his entire body was racked with sobs. I couldn't move because of the epidural. I couldn't help. I could see the neonatal NICU team and Nick resuscitating the baby, but I couldn't help. It was as if some unknown force were holding me down, for all I desperately wanted to do was . . . *Help!* my body cried out.

If I could've gotten up off the delivery table to help, I knew exactly what to do, every doctor does. Every medical student, intern, resident, and fellow does. It's called the ABCs of resuscitation and it's how we assess and treat a dying or critically injured patient. *A* is for airway—make sure you have an unobstructed airway through which you can deliver oxygen and ventilate the patient. *B* is for breathing—make sure when you are breathing for the patient (whether with an ambu bag or with a ventilator machine) that you look, listen, and feel that the respirations are expanding both lungs equally and are effective. *C* is for circulation—during this phase you need to make sure you are not only controlling any hemorrhage if it is occurring but also gaining intravenous access and assessing the patient's overall circulation. In other words, is there an adequate blood pressure to sustain life? In the multiple-injured patient, such as a motor vehicle accident, we add *D* and *E*. *D* is for deficit/disability. Does the patient have a neurologic injury? Is he conscious? *E* is for exposure—we cut off all of the patient's clothes with trauma shears to do a thorough head-to-toe exam called a secondary survey.

Because I couldn't get up to help with the ABCs, I instead did what I always do when I am scared or feel helpless: I prayed. Hail Marys always seem to work for me and give me great comfort in the quiet hours of my need. After I had whispered one or two, I heard the most beautiful of sounds—the unmistakable cry of a child. Like the peal of a church tower bell, it cut through all the other noise in the room. People shouting, monitors beeping. That crying voice gave a singular clarity to the room and said, "Our child is alive! He is healthy and alive!"

My labor had been difficult and went on for hours, which exhausted me and my then-unborn son. My obstetrician had to resort to an extended episiotomy and a vacuum-assisted delivery. I remember that last push. Nick was on my left side and was holding my lower leg, bent at ninety degrees at the knee and hip. He looked straight into my eyes and said, "Now *push!*" I will never forget that look. I have seen it many times from other surgeons across the OR table from me. It's a look you see in their eyes when a patient is bleeding out into their hands. It's a look that combines desperation, dread, and fear. All surgeons know that look. Nick and I were surgeons. We knew that look.

And so I gave it my all. I knew that our baby was in serious trouble and needed to come into the world . . . *right . . . now!*

Apgar scores have a range of 1 to 10 and are based on the overall health of a newborn after childbirth. It is a systematic evaluation of the newborn's appearance, heart rate, reflexes, muscle tone, and breathing pattern and was devised by Dr. Virginia Apgar in 1952. Our son's first Apgar was 0. *Zero!* To at least give him a 1, he had to have a heart rate. Any heart rate. He didn't even have that when he finally emerged from my body. Once he took a breath, though, a "life" switch went on in his body and all systems responded. His next Apgar was a perfect 10, and I am happy to report that I have a normal, healthy kid.

Surprisingly, getting pregnant was a lot easier than actually having the child. I was thirty-nine years old and had gone to see my OB-GYN for a routine pelvic exam. Not only was this doctor a friend of mine, but she was also the wife of one of the surgeons in my group practice. She asked me if I had thought about having children, a subject that had never really come up between us either personally or professionally. Instead of my usual answer of "never" I said, "Maybe. Sometimes." To which she responded, "You better hurry up."

It had never occurred to me that my ovaries were on a timer. As I said, I was thirty-nine years of age and felt neither old nor infertile. Every goal that I have set for myself in life I have achieved. I want to go to college. Done. I want to go to medical school. Done. I want to be a heart surgeon. Done. I want to get married. Done. I want an MBA. Done. I keep my goals simple and focused and I never predicated one on another. In other words, when it comes to goals I never engage in "if/then" thinking. "If I get this student loan, then I will go to college." Where there is a will, there is a way. And I felt the same about getting pregnant. If that is my wish, my goal, then I will achieve it. But the statistics facing women trying to get pregnant while teetering on the age of forty are frightening. According to the American Society for Reproductive Medicine, two-thirds of women in their forties have infertility problems. At age forty and older, a woman has a 5 percent chance of getting pregnant in any single ovulation

Heart Matters

cycle. Even if she does get pregnant, a forty-year-old woman will face a 24 percent miscarriage rate. And so, at last I did encounter the first "if/then" goal that I had ever faced: *If* I ovulate, *then* I will (may) get pregnant. I was at a loss as to how to handle this goal.

I had been married for two years and had been at my current job for three years. The timing seemed right, and according to my OB-GYN, Violet, I needed to "get a move on." Nick and I spent a lot of time talking about having a child. We were both scared. Neither of us pushed the other to make a decision. We made our decision to have children together. No pressure. We shared a goal between us that sprang from our love and commitment, and in that we took great comfort.

I kept the pregnancy quiet for a long time after I had successfully passed the eleven-week genetic testing known as chorionic villus sampling. I continued to take on a full workload, spending long hours standing in the OR, and even continued to fly around LA in helicopters to retrieve donor organs. Eventually, the demands of surgery and the vibrations of the helicopters caused me to have preterm labor. I was ordered on bed rest by my OB-GYN, which, for someone who goes 150 mph all the time, was no easy feat. I feared that I would lose the baby *and* my job, and I had worked so hard to have both. Women in their late thirties and forties with high-powered jobs (women I call WOP, for women of power, or CIC, for chicks in charge), please hear me loud and clear: *You can have both!* You just have to be willing to take the risk. Trust me on this. I see people die every day, and life is too short not to have it all. And that faint sound you hear in the background of your heart *is* that clock ticking. If I can do it, anyone can.

The incredible thing about being pregnant and being

a doctor is that you have so much medical insight into what is happening to your body. Did you know, for example, that your blood volume in your body increases by 50 percent during pregnancy or that your heart rate speeds up to ninety beats per minute, resulting in a 30 percent to 40 percent increase in cardiac output (the amount of blood your heart pumps per minute)? I could feel my earlobes bob to the beat of my heart as blood *whooshed* out of my left ventricle to my aorta and up my carotid arteries in my neck. The engorged veins in my hands became pipes that carried blood back to my heart, which was pumping like a Thoroughbred running a nine-month race. I remember, as a medical student, that we would be sent to the obstetrics floor to practice inserting IVs on the pregnant women because they were "easy sticks." Your body does all this in preparation for childbirth and the inevitable blood loss that occurs. Which is why women can lose so much blood during a delivery and not become anemic.

My second child, also a son, took a bit more strategy and planning but no less work or commitment to conceive, bear, and birth him. I was forty-one years old and my OB-GYN was again nudging me about "tick-tock." Since my husband and I come from large families (he has five siblings and I have four), we felt it was important for Nicholas to have a brother or sister. We also knew that by starting a family so late we would likely not be around when Nicholas was in midadulthood and we didn't want him to be alone in the world. That, and I had more than enough love in my heart for a second child. And that is how I found myself, at forty-two years of age, pregnant in the middle of my MBA at a top-ten business school.

As rigorous as the UCLA program was, it was better than

standing in the OR all day. Classes were held on Fridays and Saturdays, and the days could be twelve hours long. My strategy in class was to sit in the last row so I could be closer to the bathroom and farther from the eyes of the professor. When my legs began to swell from sitting for so long, I would prop them up on my Tumi briefcase. If I had had a drink in my hand with an umbrella in it, I'd have truly looked like I was lounging through class (although I was certainly not!). The entire academic community at the UCLA Anderson School was so supportive of my plight that they made it easy to have both—an MBA and a baby. So easy, in fact, that two other women and eleven wives of the men in my class also had babies during the twenty-three-month Executive program. With one set of twins being born, it made the total number of babies born to our class fifteen. We were one fertile group of students!

When it came to planning the birth, that was a no-brainer. I was going to have an elective caesarean section and have the baby cut out between class weekends and just after finals. This way I would miss as little class time as possible, since there were rules about how much class you could miss before your grades suffered.

The only scary incident during my second pregnancy was when, at twenty-three weeks, I had a spontaneous hemorrhage. I went to the ED for an ultrasound, thinking that I had lost the baby, but there on the ultrasound I could see it, that wonderful persistent heartbeat. We named the baby right then and there in the ED—Gabriel. He was our angel and a gift from God. His middle name, Evan, is for my aunt Evelyn, my mother's older sister, who was like a second mother to me. She had died of metastatic breast cancer on February 8, 1986, at the age of fifty-four. Our oldest son, Nicholas, we named for a long-standing tradition in my family—my dad, my eldest brother, and my husband all share that name, which makes family get-togethers at my mom and dad's house a bit confusing.

So here I am now, at forty-five, with two beautiful healthy boys who run to me with arms open wide to jump into my embrace, placing our hearts against one another, every time I come home. Can you imagine anything more wonderful or more comforting to come home to after a difficult day at work? Like any mother, I can tell you a thousand stories about the things my children do, but that might bore you. But indulge me, if you will, to tell you just one.

My husband and I make it a point to try to attend church with the children every Sunday. We organize our weekend rounds at the hospital around when the services are held because church strengthens us and nourishes our souls. It also gives us an opportunity to pray for the recovery of our patients. The boys go with us for communion to get a blessing. I had Gabriel, two years old at the time, in my arms as we approached the pastor, who was distributing the communion wafers. When we got within five people in line away from the pastor, Gabriel yelled out as loudly as his little voice could muster, "I WANT THE WHITE COOKIE! I WANT THE WHITE COOKIE!" Everyone in the church proceeded to laugh despite the solemn ceremony at hand. When we got to the chalice with wine he yelled, "IF I CAN'T HAVE THE COOKIE, THEN I WANT THE JUICE!"

As I walked back up the aisle to my pew, blushing and stifling my own laughter, I shook my head and thought, "Ya know, kids are alright."

19

Healing Robots

IT'S HARD TO EXPLAIN TO YOUR CHILDREN WHY MOMMY IS frantically searching for her socks in the middle of a calm crisp Sunday afternoon. Why she is running to her car with her sneakers in her hand. Why she is speeding off with the flashers on.

When I returned home later that day, having saved a life, I was greeted by a note on my front door from a neighbor who was "commenting" on the speed of my departure from the house. To say the note was nasty would be an understatement. I sat down at the kitchen table, noting the blood that had soaked through my canvas sneakers and onto my white ankle socks and mentally wrote an apology note to my neighbor explaining that I "just had to get to Blockbuster and pick up the latest release of *Ferris Bueller's Day Off* before the store closed."

My socks, my sneakers, and my rate of speed are immaterial to me as long as no one gets hurt. The "no one" that I am most worried about hurting, however, is my children. It is

hard for them to understand the demands of our jobs, especially when we are called away suddenly. And so my husband
and I, out of pure love for our children, have a special way of
handling the head-on collision between our work lives and
our home lives. We incorporate the kids, on some small level,
into our working world rather than isolate them from it. There
are some parents who keep their work lives entirely separate
from their home lives. When they are at work—they work.
When they are home—there is no mention of work. And the
two shall never meet. For us, this is impossible, and we have
found that making the children feel like they are a part of what
we do each day gives them the sense of belonging to part of a
greater good. They get a sense of responsibility and a sense of
control over the situation. They take ownership of what is
happening rather than being victims of it.

As an example, when my husband gets called in to do a
liver transplant in the middle of the night, it invariably wakes
up our five-year-old, Nicholas. (I could do an open heart surgery case in the middle of Gabriel's room and he wouldn't so
much as roll over in his sleep.) My husband, Nick, will take
the time to explain to Nicholas what he is doing.

"Where are you going, Daddy?"

"Well, Tiger, there is a sick patient who needs a liver
transplant tonight. Right away. I have to get on a helicopter
and go and get the liver." I believe Nicholas thinks that donor
livers come from stores and we have to fly to the store to get
them because we haven't yet told him that they come from
dead people—a bit too much for a five-year-old . . .

"What color is the helicopter?" Nicholas always wants to
know details about what's going on and I think this helps him
to picture it better in his mind.

"Blue and silver."

"Will you wear a seat belt?"

"Of course."

"Do they have snacks?"

"Sometimes."

"Tell me about the patient, Daddy." Nick will talk about the patient in terms of what he does, where he lives, and what his family is like so Nicholas can get a sense of the person and not the disease.

"What's the patient's name?" Nicholas *always* asks this.

"Jonas."

"Let's say a prayer for Jonas, Daddy."

Nick and Nicholas will say a prayer for the patient so he has a "good operation" and "feels better." So now, Nicholas knows where Daddy is going and why. He also feels like a part of the process because he believes, in a most sincere way, that his prayers will help this patient as much as Daddy's surgical skills. Nick will also follow up with Nicholas to let him know how the patient is doing each day and Nicholas is delighted about being included in Daddy's daily reports.

On weekends, especially on days like Mother's Day, when I seem to always be on call and have to make rounds (how I wish they'd invent a new holiday called Working Mother's Day specifically for moms who work so we could have the day off), I often bring the boys to the hospital with me. This delights the nurses, who then ply them with apple juice, graham crackers, and Jell-O until they "spin" from the sugar high that they never get at home.

"Don't go to work today. Mommy, please don't go." The words pierce my chest like a well-tossed javelin.

"Do you want to go with me?" I say to my sons.

"Sure." Both of their little faces light up.

We hold hands as we glide from room to room checking in on patients who are in various stages of recovery from heart surgery. I was examining the surgical incision of one particular patient when Gabriel asked, "What's that?" pointing to the man's chest. "It's his incision, honey," I replied.

"It's a crack-a-cision?" Gabriel asked.

I thought about it for a moment. Well, of course, to a three-year-old, an incision would look like a crack in the body. It was his interpretation of what he was seeing and I just went with it.

"Yes, it's his crack-a-cision."

"How come he has a crack-a-cision?"

"So he can feel better."

You could see the gears turning in his head. He was trying to figure out how a pretty nasty-looking "crack" like that could actually make a person feel better. It looks more like a very painful, yet well-placed, lethal injury. And, yes, I admit that it is a bit strange that we, as heart surgeons, can violate the human body in such a grotesque way and actually improve a patient's outcome. We heal by penetrating the chest and manipulating the core of our human physiology. How crazy is that?

When we get to intensive care, Gabriel, a little shy, just wants to "see the bones," and so I plop him down in front of the X-ray viewing machine to look at the morning's chest X-rays to his heart's content. Nicholas, more adventurous, wants to "see the patients with the zippers" (referring to my sternotomy incisions). It amazes me how this little boy will walk right up to a patient lying in an ICU bed, with nine different tubes and hoses going into and out of his body, on a ventilator, completely unconscious, and touch his hand and whisper (so he "doesn't wake him"), "Hope you feel better." He'll then smile at me proudly as if he has just cured the patient of cancer. He feels good. He feels proud. He feels like he has played a part in the patient's healing. He is not filled with fear. He is filled with hope, as in "Hope you feel better"—his own words. His own contribution.

I suppose that is how it came to pass that he started drawing "healing robots" for my patients. Nicholas loves art. Colored pens and paper are his constant companions and he is always sketching something. One morning he asked me, "Mommy, who is your sickest patient?"

"Richard," I replied. "He has water on his lungs and is very, very sick."

Nicholas made a drawing of a robot and explained to me that this was a "healing robot" and "if you put it in Richard's room, it will make him get better." And so I did. I taped it to the blank wall in Richard's room that he stared at every day, all day, and guess what? He got better.

Sometimes I feel like a healing robot—a two-dimensional piece of paper taped to a wall, not doing anything medically or surgically for patients but somehow, indirectly, helping them to get better. To heal them just by being there in their room.

"Who is your sickest patient today, Mommy?"

"Oh, Nicholas, today I have a very sick patient. Her name is Kimberly and she is a mommy. She has a son just like you, except older. He sleeps in his mommy's room at the hospital every night because he loves her so much."

Kimberly was an amazing woman who cared deeply about everyone around her and thought little of her own well-being. Riddled with metastatic cancer, she would greet me each morning by asking *me* how *I* was feeling, *I* had a lousy cold. *She* had metastatic cancer. Fluid had accumulated around her heart, known as a pericardial effusion, which had been surgically drained. Every day I would check the drainage tube that had been left in place to see how much it had drained overnight. The tube needed to be removed in order for her to go home— to go home to die. This damn tube held her hostage at the hospital because it kept draining liters of fluid.

Two days before she died, I went to see her and she did not look good at all. She was ashen, slumped in her chair and her dark, dank hair hung limp around her face. Her breathing was labored and shallow.

"How do you feel today?" she asked me as always, except that her words were more feeble and breathless.

"I feel like we should move to intensive care today, that's how I feel," I replied, which made her chuckle.

"That's a heck of an answer. Is your cold really that bad that you need to be in intensive care?"

I just smiled at her wryness. She used to be a comedian and I suppose that humor was the last vestige of her life that she had left. She had carried the torch for two blocks of its cross-country journey in the 1984 Olympics and this was the last leg of her race.

The day she moved to the ICU was the day she officially became my sickest patient on rounds. It was also the day that Nicholas drew her a healing robot. Actually, it wasn't a healing robot per se; it was a healing rainbow. Nicholas drew a beautiful picture of the sun and a rainbow. When I asked Nicholas why he drew Kimberly a rainbow instead of a robot, he replied, "Because Kimberly needs to go over the rainbow to get better." Now, mind you, Nicholas knew nothing of this woman's grave illness and the fact that she was about to die. I found that rainbow deeply prophetic.

The following morning, rainbow in one hand, Scotch tape in the other, I went to Kimberly's room in the intensive care unit. Her son was asleep on a cot next to her bed. He was wearing headphones and was breathing the soft, comfortable, evenly paced breath of someone fast asleep. Kimberly was in a rumpled hospital bed with the side rails pulled up. Her face was partially obscured by an oxygen mask. Unlike her son's breathing, her breath was agonal and came in spurts. Long, slow breaths followed by pregnant pauses. Although it was a beautiful Southern California morning, none of the day's sunlight seemed to pass through the window of Kimberly's room, although I can't quite explain why. In one corner of the room lay her and her son's personal items stuffed into four plastic hospital bags. They had simply been stacked in the corner and hadn't been put away, as if the move from her other room on the regular ward was a hurried one. Perhaps it was.

Kimberly opened one eye and, with a weary look, took notice of my taping up the picture. I told her that my son had drawn her a healing rainbow. She didn't hear me or at least didn't acknowledge she had. It didn't matter. I taped it high enough on the wall across from her bed so it would be at eye level if she opened her eyes again. She never did. As I turned to leave the room, having done nothing medically or surgically to help Kimberly, her son awoke. Half asleep, he poured himself into a chair next to the side of his mom's bed. His movements were slow and well rehearsed as if this is what he did upon waking every morning. He looked at his mom awash in sickness and tried to get closer to her by leaning over the bed rail and placing his arm around her head to cradle her in its crook. He didn't notice me standing there, the two-dimensional healing robot, doing nothing—until I spoke.

"Do you want to get in bed with your mom?" I asked.

"Is that possible?" he said, a bit bewildered.

"Everything is possible."

I called the nurse in, an exceptionally kind nurse indeed, and together she and I gently moved Kimberly to the far side of the hospital bed to make room next to her for her only son. He was a strapping young man in his twenties, yet gently, so very gently, he climbed into bed next to her.

I raised the side rail on his side of the bed, pulled the covers over the two of them, and turned out the lights. He cuddled her with both arms wrapped around her body and her head rested against his chest just the way I cuddle my sons when they sneak into my bed in the wee hours of the night.

Within three minutes of settling in next to her son, Kimberly took her last breath and died in his arms. It was as if she had waited for him to get into bed next to her before she left the earth. Although I was just a healing robot and did nothing to help this woman medically, at least I gave her that—a beautiful release from her illness, a beautiful exit from this world. When it's my time to go, that's how I want to die. In the arms of my son.

"How did Kimberly like my picture?" Nicholas asked when I got home that evening.

"She liked it very much," I replied. "And you know what she did? She went over your rainbow and is feeling much better now."

. . .

And so I say to you, working parents, involve your children in your work. Do it in a safe and nurturing way that makes them comfortable in your working world. And maybe, just maybe, they won't feel so far away from you when you're at work being a healing robot.

20

Just Breathe

M Y FAVORITE EVENT AT THE WINTER OLYMPICS IS THE biathlon. I like the fact that it is a composite event and requires equal proficiency at cross-country skiing immediately followed by riflery. I am always amazed at how the athletes can transition from the grueling energy expenditure of skiing cross-country to assuming a prone position and trying to shoot a forty-five-millimeter (1.8-inch) target fifty meters (160 feet) away with a .22LR ammo bolt action rifle.Incredible! No panting. No tremor. Just calm precision and aim while their heart rate is probably upward of 130 beats per minute.

Inhale ... .

It is the first day of school. My son Nicholas is beginning a transitional kindergarten year at a new school and, for my son Gabriel, it is his first day of preschool. It's a *big* day. I awaken at my usual predawn hour to make two healthy (no cookies, no crackers, no chips—not even Pirate's Booty—no Fruit Roll-Ups), trash-free (not even napkins), environmentally friendly contained lunches. I am in heaven. The house is quiet except for the tinkle of freshly brewed coffee dripping into the carafe, and I am relishing this work that makes me feel like a mommy. A *real* mommy. I lay out before me quite the elaborate spread of lunch materials. There will be carrots with organic dressing for dipping. There will be freshly steamed broccoli. There will be three types of cherry tomatoes that I carefully selected from the Santa Monica Wednesday-morning farmers' market. For dessert there will be sliced ripe green melon with organic cheese squares. And, of course, there will be my specialty—turkey and cheese roll-up sandwiches with mayo and broccoli sprouts. Yes, these will be the Wolfgang Puck–Martha Stewarts of lunches. I may even take a picture of them.

As I carefully place the goodies into their own distinctly shaped, hermetically sealed plastic containers, which I labeled the night before with each child's name by using one of those handheld label "guns" from Staples that punch crisp white capital letters onto a colored strip of adhesive plastic, it dawns on me that I have no idea where my husband is. Perhaps it was that I was just caught up in the lunch-making extravaganza of the first day of school. Perhaps it was the intoxicating nutty aroma of my first cup of morning coffee being brewed. Whatever the reason, it had taken me nearly thirty minutes to realize that he wasn't in the house.

Wasn't he in bed with me when I got up? No, but both kids had climbed in during the night and their two intermingled bodies under the covers could easily be mistaken for a single adult form. Let's check for the car. Nope. His car is not out front in its usual spot but he could've parked around the corner. The telltale clue that he was no longer present in the house was not the absence of a body in the bed or a car on the street but the small, unobtrusive note that I had overlooked next to the coffeepot. Written on a pink Post-it note usually reserved for the love notes that I tuck into the boys' lunches every day was scrawled the words "GSW liver." This is surgeon secret code for "gunshot wound to the liver." This could otherwise be construed for a love note of sorts between two surgeons. These eight letters told me all I needed to know about where Nick was, what he was doing, and how screwed up my day was going to be without his help getting the kids off to their first day of school.

By the way, if you are going to shoot someone in the abdomen, the place to aim is the liver because it bleeds viscously. It's not like the stomach or intestines, which, when punctured by a bullet, cause a slow death from an abdominal infection and sepsis. A GSW liver is a true surgical emergency and often very tricky to handle. A liver transplant surgeon who knows his way around the liver like he knows his way around his living room is just what you need along with some great trauma surgeons if you want to survive this lethal blow. That's my Nick.

Okay. So he's got a great excuse for missing the first day of school.

I proceed to get two handsome blond boys dressed and ready for school, and lunches in hand, we set out for an adventurous new day. Both kids are excited and a little anxious about school and I can't help but think that these are but the first steps down a path that leads to a lifetime of learning. Between my husband and me, we attended forty-three years of school and it began with that first exciting, anxious day.

At this early point in the day, I am relaxed and confident that it will all work out the way I have it planned in my head, and I had the morning off from work on this special day:

1. *Drop off Nicholas first at 9:00 a.m. and stay awhile until he is comfortable with his new teachers.*

2. *Take Gabriel to school, arriving at 9:30 a.m., and stay until noon to observe and offer support as he goes through the separation process that has been very lovingly formulated by the school.*

3. *Have my caregiver meet me at Gabriel's school at noon sharp to pick up Gabriel.*

4. *Get to the OR by 12:15 p.m. to assist my partner with a quadruple bypass case.*

5. *Hit an eyebrow waxing appointment at 5:30 p.m., which I have missed consecutively for the past three months, resulting in a unibrow.*

6. *Get home by 6:00 p.m. to make dinner and enjoy it with my family.*

Yes, I am relaxed and confident. I am so enjoying this morning, meeting the other new mommies at my son's preschool as we sit in little wooden kids' chairs neatly lined up along one wall of the classroom. I watch with pride as Gabriel is drawn to the Play-Doh and building blocks and begins to create a towering structure. He, too, is relaxed and confident in these new surroundings. Occasionally, he comes over to where I am sitting, perched in my assigned seat, to get a hug and kiss and a little reassurance about how grand this school is, but otherwise he seems quite content.

My relaxation and confidence lasts right up until the moment my caregiver calls to tell me she has a "personal emergency" and cannot meet me at the school at noon—at which point it all goes right out the window. I see my day fall into ruins, each planned event toppling like dominoes until nothing is left standing. I call Nick on the secret five-digit extension that puts me right into his OR. He is up to his elbows in hepatic arteries, portal veins, and bile ducts, so a nurse holds a phone to his ear.

"Is there any way, *any way at all,* that you can pick up Gabriel from school at noon?" I ask.

"Ummmmm . . . [*long pause*] . . . Yeah sure," Nick answers. He seems a bit distracted.

"Exactly at noon? You're sure you can do that? Because I gotta be in the OR and I mean *standing* in the OR, scrubbed, next to the operating table by twelve fifteen and that can only happen if you are here at noon on the dot."

"Gotcha. I'll be there. I'm starting to close."

"Let's have a drain," I can hear him say to the scrub nurse.

His voice cuts out as the nurse takes the phone from his ear. She forgets, however, to hang up the phone and I am left listening to the audio portion of the abdominal closure. This, however, turns out to be a wealth of information for me, because I can tell precisely where Nick is in his operation and can thus reliably predict when he will finish. Like breaking the scrambled communication code between army troops on the move, I can pinpoint his exact location in the operation, what he is doing, what his next move will be before I rendezvous with him at the school.

So now, while I try to enjoy watching Gabriel's wide-eyed

exploration of all the wonderful activities the school has to offer him on his first day, a digital clock with bright red numbers is blinking in my head: 12:15, 12:15, 12:15.

"I need the number one PDS suture" I hear Nick say through my spy cell phone, which I have concealed under my left thigh.

"Great," I think to myself. "He's closing the fascia."

Gabriel joins the circle of children on the rug.

Still blinking in my head: 12:15, 12:15, 12:15.

"I'll take a number one Prolene please."

Terrific, almost done. Just the skin left . . .

The children sing "There were five in the bed and the little one said, 'Roll over, roll over.' So they all rolled over and one fell out. There were four in the bed and the little one said . . ."

"Monocryl for the skin," I think I hear him say.

"Monocryl? They don't use Monocryl to close the skin in a trauma case. I must have heard that wrong. Staples would be faster and the closure of choice," I think out loud.

At precisely 12:02 p.m. Nick arrives to pick up a very happy Gabriel. I do a mad dash to the hospital and change into scrubs with the speed and agility of Superman in a phone booth. I take the stairs two at a time to the surgery floor, run down the hall to the OR, and almost buy it on the wet floor near the scrub sink. I scrub, dry, gown, and glove and arrive at the OR table at 12:14 p.m.! Without so much as an exhale, I calmly pick up the suture (my heart rate *easily* 130 beats per minute) and begin to sew while a single bead of sweat forms on my brow.

"How's it going?" my partner asks.

"Great," I answer in the most nonchalant tone I can muster.

Well, the rest of the day went as planned. Unibrow be gone (thanks, Keri). When we finally sat down to dinner together that night, we talked about how everyone's day went. The kids talked about their new schools, Nick talked about his case, and I, well, I simply said, "Today I did a biathlon," which my five-year-old thought was some type of heart operation. I guess, in a sense, it is.

Exhale . . .

Inhale . . .

"Just meet me on Sunset Boulevard."

"Where on Sunset Boulevard?"

"I don't know. Just start driving down Sunset and look for me. I'll be pulled off to the side of the road. And hurry, Kath, please hurry."

Nick sounded more than a little anxious . . .

Because my husband drives a large bile-green SUV with plates that read LIVER365, he's hard to miss. He had found a safe area to pull off the road on Sunset Boulevard just before the entrance to lot 4 on the UCLA campus near the Anderson School. I didn't get the whole story. There wasn't enough time. Apparently "someone" had pulled out a blood pressure monitoring catheter called an arterial line, or "art line" in medical slang, from one of his liver transplant patients, and the patient was bleeding out from the puncture site. The ICU team was holding pressure on the bleeding site and heading to the OR. Nick had to be there. Now.

The problem was, he had the kids.

He had spent a lovely summer morning with the boys at the beach, where they played in the sand and surf. They had built a few sand castles they were quite proud of, and as boys usually do, they had kicked them all down. They had also managed to fly a shark-shaped kite to the utter delight of our five-year-old, whose current passions include sharks and superheroes. And Godzilla.

So I made my way down Sunset Boulevard as fast as the turns and bends in this windy and rather dangerous road would safely allow. Anyone who has driven on Sunset can tell you that it is not the road upon which to test your brakes. When I reached Nick, I pulled over next to him and we both leapt out of our cars. Without speaking, we knew exactly what to do—transfer the kids. We each took a side of Nick's car and quickly unbuckled the car seat straps, thus freeing both boys simultaneously. I ran to my car and opened both back doors and made sure that each set of car seat straps was untangled and ready to accept both children. With child number one in hand, Nick ran around his car to my car and strapped Nicholas in. I ran around my car to Nick's car to retrieve child number two and brought Gabriel back to my car and secured him in place. Such precision and timing is seen only during a Cape Canaveral shuttle launch. To anyone passing along Sunset Boulevard that afternoon, however, we must have looked like the Keystone Kops. With a quick kiss and a "gotta go," Nick sped off to his hospital to save a life.

As I headed for home, I looked in the rearview mirror and noticed three things about my children that I hadn't during the exchange: (1) They were soaking wet, (2) they were covered in sand from head to toe, and (3) they were grinning from ear to ear. So I asked the two Cheshire cats sitting in the backseat of my car, "Why are you smiling?" "That was fun!"

they exclaimed in unison. And they were right. My life, as hectic, chaotic, and unpredictable as it can be, *is* fun. It's not dull,
I am certain of that. No offense, but can you imagine living
this life with an investment banker?

People often ask Nick and me, "How do you guys do it?"
I wish I could say that I have seven caregivers and am on Ritalin, but alas, this is not the case. I can't afford seven caregivers, and besides, Ritalin causes hand tremors that just won't
do for a cardiac surgeon. There is no singular magical formula
that makes it all work but I can tell you that communication
and flexibility are key. Nick and I talk throughout our day and
coordinate our responsibilities to each other, our children,
and our patients. We keep in contact throughout the day because things change at a moment's notice. It's the constant
tweaks and adjustments of our schedules and responsibilities
that fine-tunes everything into a dynamic balance. Who's going to go to Nicholas's school to help them make sandwiches
for the homeless? Who's going to the boys' Tae Kwon Do lesson with Master King? Who's going to take Gabriel to his 6:00
p.m. Mommy/Daddy and Me class at Saint Matthew's parish?
These are all in balance with Who's going to complete the bile
duct anastomosis on that liver transplant patient? Who's going
to run up to the cath lab and see the left main blockage that
the cardiologist can't stent? Who's going to the mandatory ad-
ministrative meeting to discuss the Women's Health Center at
their hospital?

My own personal work-life balance issues came to a head
when I decided to breast-feed my children. This single nurturing act nearly derailed me as a mother and surgeon. Coor-
dinating pumping my breast milk with my hectic operative
schedule took some serious planning and commitment, but it

was so important to me to nurse my children that I just made it work. I nursed Nicholas for eighteen months and Gabriel for a little over a year. I would have nursed them until kindergarten—that's how much I loved it! To come home at night after a grueling day and retire to the quiet comforts of the nursery. To gently rock my babies to sleep at my breast while humming "Edelweiss." To feel the soporific sway and ease of the baby-blue glider that my mother gave to me. To nuzzle their fine downy hair and indulge in their unique scent. If, when we die, we can remain forever in one moment of our lives, this would be it for me.

But trying to keep up my milk production and operate was a monumental task. I did it by making "pumping my milk" a priority each day and planned everything else around it. I owned not one, not two, but four breast pumps, some of which were hospital grade. I had an adapter that fit into the cigarette lighter in any vehicle, several electrical cords of varying lengths, and a backup battery pack to power the pump if all else failed. In case I crash-landed on a deserted island, I even had a manual pump for extreme pumping conditions. I pumped everywhere—in my office, in the locker room, in the helicopter, in an ambulance going 100 mph with lights and sirens ablaze. Yes, a lot of people got to see my breasts, but hey, they were nothing special. Sometimes I would have to leave the OR and be replaced by another surgeon for a pumping break. When the surgeons whom I was working with at the time complained, I confidently explained that I had scrubbed them out of surgery for "bathroom breaks" many times and that I, like them, was simply relieving myself of an uncomfortable bodily fluid buildup, which was just a different color than theirs. I still have an e-mail that I was once sent about how my breast-feeding was "inappropriate." I retrieve it from a file deeply embedded in my laptop named "Just for Kicks," whenever I need a good laugh.

Work-life balance is exactly what you think it is—a balance between your career and everything outside of your career. You have to decide where to place the fulcrum so that you can teeter between your work and your life without having the swings become too extreme. Because in those extremes lies all the stress imposed upon your life while out of balance. And so my advice to all of you moms who are struggling with home and career responsibilities is that each morning you should wake up and set your priorities for the day. And only that day, taking one day at a time. Look for the trade-offs that you have to make and that is where your fulcrum lies. Then balance each responsibility against the other in order of priority. Oh, and don't forget to call your partner and fill him in on the details of the day.

It's like a deliciously tossed salad with just the right amount of love, respect, communication, and flexibility. And sure, you don't always get the ingredients just right, but it is a delicacy to be savored just the same. And everyone, no matter how crazy you think your life is, can enjoy a taste. The bitter and the sweet.

Exhale . . .

21

Pressure

MY DAY STARTED WITH AN AUTOPSY. COFFEE, A PROTEIN shake, and an autopsy. A shower was a moot point because I'd be smelling like death all day, anyway.

I had started to make my way to the morgue when I realized that I had no idea where it was. I just assumed it was in the basement. It's *always* in the basement, as if it's the hospital's best-kept secret, as if they don't want anyone to know what's going on there. It is the hospital's very own Manhattan Project—secretive, necessary, and a very important part of the hospital's everyday working environment. I had never been to the morgue at this, my new hospital, and that is a good thing.

It's not that I hate the morgue. I just don't like going there. If I go there, it means someone has died. My patient has died. And I have failed. I am a failure. I am inadequate, inept. How can that be when I have spent my whole life trying to be successful? Trying to save life, not end it. If I fail, they fail. Our bodies and souls linked together by the same fate. I am afraid of failure. I am afraid. Me. Tough guy. Afraid.

I stepped onto the elevator. It was quiet. Deathly quiet. It was the wee morning hours and the only other person in sight was an unshaven custodian, shirt untucked, leaning on his mop next to the open elevator door. Not working. Not mopping. Just leaning. A sentinel. A guardian of the elevator. The elevator that would take me down. To the morgue. Where my day would begin with an autopsy.

I kept my head bowed, looking at my white leather sneakers and noticing a few droplets of blood. His blood. The guy in the morgue's blood. I could feel the apprehension build in my throat. The coffee-protein mixture was churning in my stomach. I kept fingering my stethoscope, an object of familiarity to me, which was in the left pocket of my wrinkled doctor's coat. The smoothness of its black finish comforted me somehow.

I didn't want to do it. I didn't want to go. I could feel that janitor looking at me, wondering what the hell I was doing standing motionless and alone in an elevator with the door open. Locked in purgatory. Neither going up nor going down. At a standstill. At a crossroad. If I went up, I would go and make rounds on the fourth floor and see my live patients. If I went down, well, you know where I'd go. To see him. The dead guy. The guy who was doing so well after surgery and was going home on Saturday. Home to his apartment, where his best friend would see him through the remainder of his recovery. But something unexplainable went wrong, horribly wrong. And the autopsy, hopefully, would tell me why. That's why I had to go and see this through. I needed to know. The devil is in the details. That red guy, the color of blood, with his trident sticking in my neck chiding me. The details. The details of an autopsy.

I clenched my back teeth together, grinding them to the point of causing a painful spasm in my jaw, swallowed hard, and pushed the down button.

The elevator lurched twice and then slowly and precariously descended. It felt like a deep dive. A decompression dive. The kind of scuba dive where they hang tanks of varying concentrations of nitrogen and oxygen at different depths to allow you to "off-gas" and rid your body of absorbed inert gases that you accumulated while diving to a depth of greater than 130 feet. I could feel the pressure surrounding me, weighing down on me. Squeezing me on all sides. My head exploding. I needed to equalize my ears, to feel the *pop!* as my Eustachian tubes opened and allowed air into or out of my middle ear, adjusting the pressure across my eardrum. Just when the pressure seemed unbearable, the elevator abruptly stopped. The door didn't open immediately, leaving me to stand there examining my full-length reflection in the chrome. The lines around my eyes and the smudged mascara beneath my lower lashes made me look so tired. So defeated. My scrubs were rumpled as if I had slept in them. My coat was wrinkled and filthy as if I had rolled around in a parking lot. I was a mess.

My first thought, of course, was "I am trapped." I am not claustrophobic, so the setting didn't really bother me except for the fact that I was stuck looking at myself. It did, however, seem a bit eerie to be trapped in the basement so close to the morgue. My life is one continual nonstop movement and I hate to stand still because I see it as an awful waste of time. To my relief, the doors creaked open slowly, grinding their edges against the metal framing. Alfred Hitchcock himself couldn't have directed the scene any better.

I stepped out of the elevator and paused. There was a stale lingering smell, the odor of wet sleeping bags. To my right was a long corridor that dead-ended into a puke-yellow painted brick wall. The hallway was empty save for a few thin, careworn ghosts in flowing garments trying to find their way out and a single steel gurney with a thick brown plastic drape that hung to the floor skirting all four sides. Every hospital has one of these seemingly innocuous gurneys. They are singular in purpose—to transport dead bodies, undercover, to the morgue. When a patient dies in the hospital in the middle of a pale blue afternoon, we put their bodies in a secret chamber below the gurney that is hidden beneath the drapes. Like some ghastly magician's vanishing act, we hide the body from the audience and simply wheel the dead patient right through the hallway. This is so that you, the loving granddaughter strolling through the hall on the way to visit your seventy-one-year-old grandmother who just had her adrenal gland removed because it contained a pheochromocytoma (a rare tumor), will not be reminded that people die in the hospital on pale blue afternoons.

To my left, the corridor was much shorter and jogged to the right. At the end of the corner there was a small, barely readable sign. The sign was yellow and blended in with the wall except for a slight contrast in hue. A remnant of a tattered toe tag rested against the cracked baseboard on the floor beneath it. With my eyes squinted, I could just barely make out the sign's lettering. CAUTION: FORMALDEHYDE, it read. Since they don't put signs like this outside the hospital boiler room, I knew in which direction the morgue lay and felt the pressure build again. I turned left.

I reached the door to the morgue. There was no sign next to it that announced WELCOME TO THE MORGUE. YOU'VE FINALLY

FOUND IT, although there should be to make people feel a little more comfortable. So how did I know this was the morgue? Because of the door. It had no handle. Just a metal push plate. It was on hinges that allowed it to swing to and fro, which enables the door to give way when an attendant, pushing a gurney, is wheeling a body into, and subsequently out of, the morgue. It would be awkward if the attendant had to turn a doorknob, open the door, and then hold it open with his foot as he maneuvered the clumsy gurney through the portal. The situation is awkward enough without having to fuss with the door.

I held my breath, let the tide of pressure wash over me, and gently pushed the door open. The smell of formaldehyde hit me right in the face. Like a bat to the bridge of the nose. I felt my face crack in three places. I blinked as the formaldehyde stung my eyes. When I could finally open my eyes without blinking, I saw that they had started without me, which pissed me off, but I said nothing. The pathologist, a shaggy young guy, was hunched over the open chest. His grim henchman assistant held the chest plate back, a technique loosely known as popping the hood, to yield exposure. "Why didn't you go through my incision?" I asked. "Because we always use the Y incision," he answered, without looking up. A Y-shaped incision runs from both shoulders to the midchest and then straight down the abdomen. It's crude but effective in giving maximum exposure to the body cavities. I observed while the pathologist inspected my work. He pointed to a few structures and asked a few questions. Then he just chopped out the heart with a large blunt pair of scissors, which hacked at the connecting structures that held the heart in place—the left internal mammary artery graft that I had labored over, the aorta, the pulmonary artery, the superior vena cava, the inferior vena cava, and the left atrium. I bit my lower lip. It hurt to see all of my effort ripped from the chest. He brought the heart to a separate table. He gave it its own space, a place of reverence and respect, so we could focus our full attention on the heart and not be distracted by any of the other vagabond structures in the chest.

We inspected each of my bypass grafts and their connections to the aorta and native coronary arteries. Every suture line was intact. We then looked at each cannulation site where the tubing from the heart-lung machine circuit was placed and removed. Each site had been reinforced with additional sutures as is my paranoid habit because a leak from one of these sites would be deadly. They were all intact. No broken sutures. No holes. My surgery had been a technical success and I felt the pressure lift just a little. A feather lifted from atop the pile of river rock stacked upon my chest.

The autopsy continued with the inspection of the other chest structures. The pathologist found a large pulmonary embolism, which had ultimately killed the patient. A sizable blood clot had traveled from its perch from within a vein in the lower body through two chambers in the heart and made a new home for itself, lodged within the pulmonary artery. The embolism prevents blood from going to the lungs so no oxygen can be delivered. The pressure builds up in the heart rapidly and can kill its victim within seconds. This is often the cause when people die in their sleep—a large blood clot that takes a northerly trip in complete silence. Without pain. Without warning, even to a physician. Leaving you, the patient, dead. A simple victim of pressure.

I wanted to spend the rest of the day sitting in my office

staring at a blank wall. I thought the autopsy would make me feel vindicated. I thought I would have closure, maybe even a little peace. I didn't.

Just as I settled into my chair, my phone rang. It was my husband. "Where are you?" Nick said. "We're almost ready." I had completely forgotten that we were supposed to meet at the house at eleven o'clock for a special event. A lasting moment. I sped from the hospital. Heart pounding. Hands gripping the steering wheel. I strategically chose the streets with the least number of traffic lights so as to shave a few seconds from my race to get home. I was flying as much as the speed limit would allow. Maybe I'd get there in time. Maybe . . . Maybe . . .

. . .

I pushed down hard on the wet cement. I put all of my weight behind it and applied a serious amount of pressure. Pushing, pushing until my wrists hurt. When I lifted my hands, I realized that I was too late. I had missed it—the one chance to make a lasting impression. The one chance to be immortalized with my family as one complete unit with our handprints. How many more moments would I miss because I am so wrapped up in my job? How many Tae Kwon Do belt testings? How many soccer games? How many Mommy and Me classes? How many good-night kisses?

My handprint was barely there in the gray concrete because it was almost dry when I finally got my hands on it. No matter how much pressure I applied, I couldn't make an impression because the cement was hardening quickly beneath my hands and I was no match for it. Even though I took all of the pressure from my day—the elevator, the morgue, my deceased patient—and channeled it from my core down my

arms and into my hands, the imprint that I left was barely visible. My husband's strong handprints, then the small awkward
prints of my sons, were clearly visible. There was a blank
space where my handprints should logically go in the family
order. Mine were missing. I was missing.

And so I sat down beside our new cement driveway and
cried. I let the tears just pour from my eyes and roll down my
cheeks. I felt them reach my jawline and then just leap off
my face onto the grayness below. I cried for the blood on my
sneakers, for the hinged breastplate, for the dismembered
heart, for the death of my patient. I cried for my hands, which
are my tools, and their weakness in making an impression that
could barely be felt in the otherwise smooth cement and not
clearly seen.

"Why are you crying, sweetie?" my husband asked. I
didn't answer. The answer was too complicated and would
suck too much energy from me.

He looked at the cement driveway and then at me. "We'll
just do it over again. A do-over. Okay? We'll just jackhammer
it out and repour it."

"A do-over," I repeated.

I nodded and got up wearily from the ground. I walked
back to my car, shoulders hunched, and drove back to work
to stare at a wall.

When I arrived back at the hospital, a thin dusting of cement still lingering on my hands, the first person I encountered
was one of my favorite nuns. The nuns are a constant loving
presence in our hospital, which was originally founded by the
Sisters of Charity of Leavenworth. Several of the nuns of this order live in a convent on the top floor of the medical center,
where they pray daily for the patients and the staff. And, yes, it
really works.

Every nun at my hospital is my favorite, really; each is special in her own unique way. Sister Maureen, however, was as much a part of the hospital as the walls themselves. And, like the walls, she held up the medical center and its doctors with her prayers, love, and support. This was her calling. She sped toward me in her wheelchair because she could clearly see my burden from a distance. I knelt down next to her so that she could look down upon me and get a better view into my soul without craning her neck. She held my hands in hers, taking no notice of their powdery cement coating. She didn't ask me what was wrong. She didn't need to. I wanted a formal blessing from her. A prayer. But instead she said with her wry Arkansas humor, "My mom used to say that when we all get to heaven, we're gonna be so surprised at God's poor taste—he lets everyone in."

And just like that, the pressure lifted.

Completely.

Finally.

EPILOGUE

I AWOKE ON THE LAST DAY OF THE YEAR A LITTLE SAD-dened by its passing. What is it about time that makes it seem to pass so swiftly? Time. A precious entity that can be both fleeting and simultaneously stretched to eternity. Time. It can slip right through your fingers in a heartbeat or two. Time. How we sometimes take it for granted instead of treating it like the gift it is.

My life's work has been about giving people time. Time to live and, when it is their time, time to die. I have spent a lifetime learning how to be a good surgeon, a good doctor, a good person, and I am still learning, with each passing day, how to be a good wife, a good friend, and a good mother. It all just takes time.

That morning, an enticing sound greeted me. It sounded like someone shuffling two decks of cards together. *Ratta tatta tat. Ratta tatta tat.* The sound would stop for a moment and then begin again. I went downstairs to investigate. Following the sound led me to the picture window at the front of our house where I could see the orange dawn break in the sky above the churning gray ocean. There, a tiny hummingbird furiously beat its wings against the pane of glass in the morning light. *Ratta tatta tat.* Magnificent, its iridescent feathers flickered green and blue as it hovered. Its ruby throat pulsed as its thin needle beak tapped the glass in an avian Morse code. Since hummingbirds spend 80 percent of their lives perched, I could see that this little fellow was tiring quickly.

I didn't know how to get the bird out of the house. He wasn't near a window that opened. I thought perhaps I could trap it against the window with a plastic container, cover the top with a piece of cardboard, and then carry the imprisoned bird to the front door and set it free. I worried, though, that I would harm its wings if I tried to do this. Something told me to just approach the bird gently and offer my hand, the way I have greeted a thousand patients, with kindness and compassion. A gesture of sincerity that says "I want to help you." And so I did. Slowly, steadily. I held out my index finger to the little dervish and said softly, "I won't hurt you. You are safe and I will set you free."

To my utter amazement he lit upon my finger and just sat there. I felt his body pulsate rapidly with the beat of his heart, a heart incidentally that is no bigger than a cranberry and takes up nearly 20 percent of his body volume—higher than any other animal. A heart that beats 500 times per minute while perched on my finger and can spike up to 1,200 times per minute in flight. A heart that will beat 4.5 billion times in this creature's lifetime.

I slowly walked to the front door, the door through which I pass every morning. The door that takes me away

from my family and returns me to them safely. My feet shuf-
fled smoothly along the oak flooring in a gliding motion. I
steadied my hand as I would in surgery so as not to frighten
this little interloper. He rode with me very calmly, looking at
me with his head slightly cocked to one side. It gave him a
wry appearance. Ever so gently, I reached with my free hand
and quietly opened the door, letting in the warm sunlight and
salty air. He didn't leave me immediately as I had thought he
would. He just sat there as I walked outside to the front landing. "You are free now, you can go," I said. Still, he waited a
minute more to leave. A minute that seemed to stretch time
into a moment. And then, in a hush, he lifted off and was gone
in a heartbeat.

· · ·

There are many Native American legends that surround these
tiny birds. One is that hummingbirds are believed to act as in-
tercessors between nature and the spirit world. Perhaps this
dawn visitation was from a dear friend who died recently from
cancer and came back to check in on me. Or perhaps it was a
visit from one of the departed in this book. Either way, it was
a welcome interlude indeed.

Life, like time, is precious and sometimes very short.

Let your heart race.

Let your heart soar.

Let your heart be free.

For you are only given one heart, so please take good
care of it.

Your heart matters . . .

ACKNOWLEDGMENTS

HOW DO YOU TAKE A CARDIAC SURGEON AND MAKE HER into an author? With a lot of help, support, and encouragement, that's how.

First and foremost, I would like to thank my husband, Nick Nissen, MD, without whom I could never have written this book. He is my soul mate, my friend, my confidant, and my number one supporter. He is also the most incredible physician and surgeon, whose skill, kindness, and compassion have always been an example to me. This amazing man loves me truly and believes in me in a way that gives me the strength to accomplish all of the things in my life. He has stood by me in difficult times. Times of doubt. Times of fear. Times of frustration. And he has given me the most incredible gift of all: our children.

I would also like to thank the entire Magliato clan for all of their love and support throughout my entire life. My mom, Dottie, and dad, Nick. My sister, Nancy. My brothers: Nick,

Paul, and David. My in-laws, Cristin, Jenifer, and Mark; and my nieces and nephews, Ben, Brittni, Bryant, Chris, Emme, Eric, Matt, PJ, Samantha, and Tenea.

To my friends: Donna Dubrow, for our Westlake Village Four Seasons Hotel writing retreat weekends. Tim Misenhimer, for the use of his inspirational Palm Springs home. Chavez Ransom (Uncle C), for helping Nick watch the kids so I could write. Marc Daniels, who introduced me to Robin McGraw, who said to me during highlights (and lowlights), "You should write a book," thus planting the seed in my head. Jack Grapes, for teaching me to "write like you talk."

To my colleagues, old and new: Manny Estioko, MD; Sharo Raissi, MD; John M. Robertson, MD; and John Stoneburner, MD; as well as Stephen Ritterbush, Ph.D.; and Michael Whitt, Ph.D.; and MBA at Cordex Systems, LLC, for giving me the space in my busy life to write this and for encouraging me to do so.

And to all of the professors, attendings, nurses, fellows, residents, and medical students who have taught me the art and craft of being a surgeon as well as all of the academic institutions and medical centers that have furthered my education and enhanced my practice—Union College, Albany Medical Center, Case Western Reserve University, Akron General Medical Center, Loyola University Medical Center, the University of Pittsburgh Medical Center, the University of Michigan Medical Center, the UCLA Anderson School of Management, Saint John's Hospital, and Torrance Memorial Medical Center.

I would also like to thank the following nonprofit organizations for continuing to build awareness concerning heart disease in women: The American Heart Association, Events of the Heart, Mended Hearts.

It has been my dream to write this book, and it took the sincere dedication and effort on the part of my publishing agent, Dan Strone at Trident Media, to realize that dream. The book was born during coffee at the Beverly Wilshire Hotel two years ago when Dan had the insight to turn a book about heart disease in women into a new genre that is both prescriptive and memoir. I am so grateful for the confidence he had in me, a novice writer, to tell my story.

I would also like to thank my editors, Diane Salvatore and Vanessa Mobley, at Broadway Books for the incredible opportunity to publish this work and for giving my voice a home within its pages.

Last, I would like to thank all of my patients—past, present, and future—for allowing me the honor of touching their hearts.

APPENDIX 1

Heart Disease by the Numbers

♥ 41,000,000: the number of women currently living with cardiovascular disease

♥ 8,000,000: the number of women today who have a history of having a heart attack or angina or both

♥ 5,000,000: the number of women hospitalized each year for cardiovascular disease

♥ 500,000: the number of women who die each year from cardiovascular disease

♥ 270,100: the estimated number of annual U.S. cancer deaths in women for *all* cancers combined*

♥ 213,000: the number of women who die each year from a heart attack

* All material in this chapter, except as noted, is based on D. Lloyd-Jones et al. Heart disease and stroke statistics 2009 update: a report from the American Heart Association Statistics Committee and Stroke Statistics Subcommittee, *Circulation* 119 (2009): e21–e181. National Center for Health Statistics, Deaths: Leading causes for 2004. *National Vital Statistics Reports* 56, no. 5 (2007): 1–96.

♥ 160,000: the number of women who die each year from congestive heart failure

♥ 40,480: the number of women who died from breast cancer in 2008*

♥ 58%: the percentage of women with a cholesterol level greater than 200 mg/dl

♥ 28%: the percentage of women with a cholesterol level greater than 240 mg/dl

♥ 50%: the percentage of women over the age of 55 who have high blood pressure

♥ 50%, 64%, 60%, 53%: the percentage of Caucasian, African American, Hispanic, and Asian/Pacific Islander women who lead a sedentary lifestyle, respectively

♥ 58%, 78%, 73%: the percentage of Caucasian, African American, and Hispanic women who are overweight, respectively

♥ 30%: the percentage for increased risk of heart disease with exposure to secondhand smoke

♥ 21%: the percentage for increased risk of heart disease in women who smoke and take birth control pills

♥ 38%: the percentage of women who will die within 1 year of a recognized heart attack

♥ 35%: the percentage of women heart attack survivors who will have another heart attack within 6 months

♥ 46%: the percentage of women heart attack survivors who will be disabled with heart failure within 6 months

* American Cancer Society, 2007–2008 *Facts & Figures.*

♥ 33%: the percentage of angioplasties, stents, and bypass surgery that women receive compared to men despite the fact that more women than men die each year from heart disease

♥ 28%: the percentage of women, compared with men, who receive defibrillators

♥ 27%: the percentage of women participants in all heart-related research studies

♥ 7,095,000: the number of cardiovascular operations and procedures performed in 2006, 3,100,000 of which were performed on women (yet more women than men die from heart disease each year)

♥ $475,300,000,000: the direct and indirect costs of cardiovascular disease in 2009

APPENDIX 2

How to Avoid "Going Under the Knife"

Know Your Numbers

I want you to be able to rattle off the following numbers the way you can rattle off your Social Security number. If you know them, you will own them. You must strive to keep them in the normal ranges provided.*

Blood Pressure	< 120/80 mmHg
Total Cholesterol	< 200 mg/dl
Good Cholesterol (HDL)	> 60 mg/dl
Bad Cholesterol (LDL) for high-risk women[†]	< 100 mg/dl
Bad Cholesterol (LDL) for low-risk women[‡]	< 160 mg/dl

* National Cholesterol Education Program guidelines.
[†] High-risk women defined as those who already have coronary artery disease, diabetes, abdominal aortic aneurysm, carotid artery atherosclerosis, peripheral vascular disease, or two or more risk factors for cardiovascular disease.
[‡] Low-risk women are defined as those with zero to one risk factor for cardiovascular disease.

Triglycerides	< 150 mg/dl
BMI (Body Mass Index)*	< 25
Waist Circumference	< 35 inches

FOR DIABETICS

♥ Check your blood sugar (glucose) four times daily: before each meal and at bedtime. Keep a log of these numbers to show your doctor.

♥ Your fasting blood sugar level should be < 100 mg/dl.

♥ Have your hemoglobin A1c, a measure of how well your blood sugar has been controlled, checked every 3–4 months. Normal is < 7.0.

Know Your Symptoms

Women's symptoms of heart disease differ dramatically from men's. Half of all women do not get chest pain. Here are the most common symptoms women report:

♥ Fatigue (the most common symptom of heart disease in women)

♥ Left-arm pain

♥ Jaw pain

♥ Neck/throat pain

♥ Indigestion

♥ Nausea

* BMI is calculated by dividing your weight in kilograms by the square of your height in meters (kg/m^2).

♥ Shortness of breath

♥ Light-headedness

WHAT TO DO IF YOU DEVELOP THESE SYMPTOMS

♥ Stop what you are doing.

♥ Call 911. Do *not* drive yourself to the hospital.

♥ Take your prescribed medication, which may include nitroglycerin tablets.

♥ Take a baby aspirin (81 mg) unless you have a contraindication to aspirin.

♥ Do *not* ignore your symptoms!

ABOUT THE AUTHOR

KATHY E. MAGLIATO, MD, is currently the director of women's cardiac services at Saint John's Health Center in Santa Monica, California. She lives in Pacific Palisades with her husband and their two children.